COPYRIGHT © 2024 Philippa Bebbington

All rights reserved. No part of this book may be reproduced or transmitted in any form or by any means, electronic or mechanical, including photocopying, recording, or by an information storage and retrieval system - except by a reviewer who may quote brief passages in a review to be printed in a magazine or newspaper - without permission in writing from the publisher.

The author of this book does not dispense medical advice or prescribe the use of any technique as a form of treatment for physical, emotional, or medical problems without the advice of a physician, either directly or indirectly. The intent of the author is only to offer information of a general nature to help you in your journey for emotional, physical, and spiritual well-being. In the event you use any of the information in this book for yourself, the author, and publisher assume no responsibility for your actions.

First edition, September, 2024

ISBN: 9798336930801

Disclaimer:

The information provided in this book, Cracking The Food Code: Stop Diets That Don't Work. Reboot Your Health & Habits, is for educational and informational purposes only. It is not intended to serve as medical advice or a substitute for professional consultation, diagnosis, or treatment. Always seek the guidance of your physician, dietitian, or other qualified health providers with any questions you may have regarding your health, medical conditions, or before starting any new dietary or exercise regimen.

The author and publisher of this book are not responsible for any adverse effects or consequences resulting from the use or application of any information contained in this book. The success of any nutritional or fitness program depends on the individual's commitment, diligence, and adherence to the recommendations provided. Results may vary, and individual outcomes are not guaranteed.

In addition, the information in this book may not apply to all individuals and should be tailored to meet your specific needs and circumstances. If you have any health concerns or preexisting conditions, it is important to consult with your healthcare provider before implementing any of the strategies or recommendations discussed.

By reading this book, you acknowledge and agree that the author and publisher are not liable for any actions taken by you in reliance on the information provided herein. Your health is your responsibility, and it is essential to make informed choices that are best suited for your individual well-being.

Copyright 2024 Philippa Bebbington

Published in the United States By Amazon Publishing

All rights reserved

Book design by Kim Johnson

To my beloved daughters, who inspire me every single day to be the best version of myself—for you, I strive to reach new heights and never give up. My deepest wish is that you always recognize your immense value and strength, and carry compassion and grace in all that you do. Your laughter and love are the heartbeat of my motivation, driving me to push boundaries and chase dreams.

And to my husband, my rock, thank you for your unwavering support and for encouraging me to pursue my passion with all my heart. Your unwavering dedication and deep compassion for your patients inspire me to provide my clients with the most sincere and heartfelt care I can offer.

It's the love and support of my family that has fueled this journey, turning life's challenges into opportunities, and lemons into lemonade. For this, I will forever be grateful.

Xo

Contents

Foreword by Dr. Scott Eisenberg————————————————6

A Message From The Author ————————————————10

Introduction: DIETS DON'T WORK—Spoiler Alert! ————————12
    Why Diets Fail
    The Journey Begins

Chapter 1: Cracking The Food Code ————————————--16
    The REBOOT: Your Path to Lasting Change
    Getting Started: Laying the Foundation
        RESET: Clearing the Slate
        REFUEL: Nourishing Your Body Right
        REWIRE: Transforming Your Habits

Chapter 2: Basic Nutrition 101 ————————————— 24
    Inflammation and INFLAMMAGING: What You Need to Know
    Gut Health & The Immune System: The Role of Prebiotics,
    Probiotics, & Fiber
    Water and Hydration: What's the Big Deal?
    Intermittent Fasting: Timing Your Way to Better Health

Chapter 3: Getting Started————————————— 48
    The Power of Mindset: A Message From Kim Johnson
    Tracking Your Progress on the REBOOT: Stay on Course
    Document Your Progress & Cultivate Gratitude in Your Daily
    Life
    Strategies To Enhance Gratitude: Tools for Success

Chapter 4: Cracking The Food Code—The RESET————— 58
    Days 1-21: Meat & Alcohol RESET
    Days 4-21: The Sugar RESET
    Days 7-21: Refined Fats and Oils RESET
    Days 10-21: Gluten, Grains & Inflammation—The GRAIN-
    FREE RESET
    Days 13-21: The Caffeine RESET
    Days 16-21: The Dairy RESET
    Days 19-21: The Toxin RESET: Are You Ready To Clean Up
    Your Health?

Chapter 5: REFUEL—Optimize Your Health with Balanced Nutrition and Key Supplements——— 103

Step 1: Reintroduce with Awareness—Rediscover Foods Mindfully

Step 2: Design Your Anti-Inflammatory Plan—Build Your Personalized Eating Plan

Step 3: Cleanse Your Environment—Minimize Toxins, Maximize Health

Step 4: Assess Your Nutrient Needs—Supplement Wisely, Thrive Fully

Chapter 6: REWIRE—Mastering the Art of Self-Care——— 115

Exercise and Movement: The Key to Longevity

Sleep: Recharge Your Life

Stress Management: Finding Calm in the Chaos

Overview: Wrapping Up the REWIRE

Chapter 7: Phil's 30-Day REBOOT——— 128

You've Cracked The Food Code—What's Next?

Phil's 30-Day REBOOT: Your Next Big Step to Lasting Change

The Reboot Guide ——— 133

Anti-Inflammatory Pantry Staples

Baking Staples

Breakfast Recipes

Lunch Recipes

Dinner Recipes

Sweet Treats

High Protein Snack Ideas

Grab-and-Go Healthy Snacks

Cracking the Food Code for Unimaginable Sustained Health and Wellbeing
Forward by Dr. Scott Eisenberg, DO, FACC

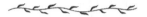

Here you are—another day of work, another day of life. At 6 am, or whenever your alarm goes off, you're faced with choices. In that moment, what is your mindset? You can choose to make decisions that will impact your lifetime or stick with the same old habits. We all know the definition of insanity, right? Doing the same thing over and over, especially when it comes to your health, wellness, and longevity, while expecting different results is, well, insane!

Yes, life is hard. But you can choose "your" hard. We all face setbacks and get knocked down. But when you're down, if you can look up, you can always get up. This is your time to get up. In a snowball fight, you have three options: duck and run for cover, stand there and keep getting hit, or throw snowballs back! It's time to start throwing. When it comes to your health, it's not just about winning—it's about being committed. The latter will always be the best path for you. Simply taking medications versus truly working on your health every single day, combining proper nutrition and exercise—this is the way to win. Being committed to being the healthiest you can be is the real victory.

Let's face it—it's not the doctor's fault, and it's not the patient's fault. It's the approach that has been failing us. The system has let us down on so many levels when it comes to helping people succeed. It's taken you years to get where you are, and for many, it's not a good place. The knowledge out there is often inaccurate or downright harmful. And as I often tell my patients, "Women and men aren't from Mars and Venus —we're from different galaxies." There are clear gender differences when it comes to weight loss, exercise, nutrition, and medications. Women are often at a disadvantage from the start, with hormone imbalances and inflammation taking over early, leaving them frustrated and searching for answers—some of which are useless or unhealthy. For men, while they tend to lose more weight and improve their risks with interventions like this, they also tend to be less compliant or drop out of the game of life more often than women.

In my 28 years of practicing cardiology, I'm still amazed at how often, when I review my patients' labs and discuss their poorly controlled blood pressure, weight, cholesterol, and blood sugar levels—and the looming risks of heart disease, stroke, and kidney failure—their immediate response is, "Can't you just give me the shot or pill?" The reluctance to embrace lifestyle changes is all too common. Unfortunately, many healthcare professionals often take the easier route, prescribing medications without first emphasizing the crucial protocol of "doing the work"—making necessary lifestyle adjustments. This goes against decades of medical guidelines that mandate trying lifestyle changes before resorting to medication (unless it's life-threatening, of course).

But it's not entirely the patient's fault. Many have tried countless diets that just don't work, leaving them feeling frustrated and defeated. They haven't been given the right tools to succeed, and without those tools, it's no wonder motivation wanes. This book offers exactly what's been missing—the tools needed to do the work, either before medication or alongside it.

The reason I know this, is because I was one of these patients...

Even as a doctor, I found myself in the same shoes as many of my patients. Two years ago, staring down the barrel of turning 60, I wasn't thrilled with what I saw in the mirror or how I felt. Embarrassingly, I, too, asked for a prescription for "the shot." But, I was told I wasn't overweight enough, diabetic enough, or had significant heart disease to qualify for coverage. So, there I was with a choice: pay for the shot out of pocket or DO THE WORK. My dietitian was absolutely livid (and for the record, she's also my wife and the author of this book). She insisted I follow her reboot protocol and actually do the work. I was skeptical—who wouldn't be? This approach was unlike anything I'd seen or even recommended to my patients before.

Admitting she was right wasn't easy (and yes, I'm putting that in writing for all eternity), but I'm glad I did. Within three weeks, I began to see real changes. My belly started to flatten, my waistline shrank, my blood pressure improved, my joint pain vanished, and I was sleeping like a baby! Fast forward seventeen months, and new patients often remark, "You look so different from your online picture." Well, that's because that picture was 40 pounds ago! I had to walk the talk I'd been preaching to my patients for years—and, more importantly, I had to listen to my dietitian (and trust me, that wasn't the easiest pill to swallow!).

Bottom line...
There's no magic bullet. If you think that simply putting a chemical in your body is winning, you've lost before you even started. Winning is about fighting, pushing, and giving it

everything you've got. Winning is moving forward. Just by picking up this book and reading it, you've already made progress.

A RESET system like this is a gift for a lifetime. We all have busy lives—work stress and life stress. We all fall back to comfort food, drink too much alcohol, and do not get nearly enough exercise when things get tough. We all play, and some of us play harder than we work. We need something we can go back to time and time again when we stray from our goals.

That's why this book is such an essential starting point. By diving into these pages, you are equipping yourself with the knowledge and strategies you need to finally take control of your health. But if you're ready to take it even further, consider pairing what you have learned in this book with the companion program, Phil's 30-Day REBOOT (you can learn more in Chapter 7). Together, they provide a sustainable, reproducible, and reliable system!

As I have said daily for the past 28 years: "Get to it before it gets to you."

To your health and happiness,
Dr. Scott R. Eisenberg, DO, FACC
Board-certified in General and Interventional Cardiology 1997-present
Certifications in both Lipidology and Anti-aging and Regenerative Medicine

A Message From The Author

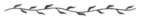

Hi, I'm Philippa Bebbington, but please, call me "Phil." I'm absolutely thrilled to welcome you here! Before we dive into "Cracking The Food Code and the secret to REBOOTING your health," let me formally introduce myself.

I proudly juggle a lot of hats each day—I'm a mom to two amazing daughters (one's a physician assistant, and the other is a registered nurse), a supportive wife to an interventional cardiologist, a stepmom to three wonderful kids, and a dedicated pet parent to both dogs and a cat. Oh, and I'm also a Registered Dietitian and Integrative Health Coach. Like so many of us, I got used to balancing these roles, but it was this very balancing act that propelled me on my own journey toward self-healing.

The REBOOT program started out as a deeply personal project, but it's not just about me—it's about you. It's about helping people like you take back control of their health and well-being through smart nutrition and lifestyle changes. The foundation of Phil's REBOOT is Bioindividuality—the understanding that there's no one-size-fits-all approach to health. Diets often fail because we're all unique, and our bodies respond differently to various foods and lifestyles. This program is here to teach you how to RESET your metabolism, REFUEL your body with nutrition tailored to your needs, and REWIRE your mindset around food and health.

I'm genuinely excited to see the incredible progress you'll make on your journey to optimal health. Remember, this is all about progress over perfection", so be kind to yourself along the way.

With commitment and effort, the rewards will be more than worth it. I can't wait to see the amazing transformations you're going to achieve!

With Love,

Phil

Introduction

DIETS DON'T WORK!

Let's be honest: Americans have a bit of a love affair with diets. According to Harvard Health, at any given moment, about one-third of Americans are on a specific diet, usually aiming for weight loss. But it doesn't stop there—plenty of people are also dieting to lower cholesterol, manage diabetes, control autoimmune diseases, ease menopausal symptoms, and more. Sounds great in theory, right? The problem is, while these diets might deliver some impressive short-term results, keeping those results over the long haul is like trying to keep a toddler from eating crayons—nearly impossible! Research shows that most of the health benefits from diets tend to vanish after a year, sometimes even sooner.

And then there's the new craze: weight loss and blood sugar medications—the so-called "magic pills" or shots. It's tempting, isn't it? The promise of maximum results with minimal effort is a siren call that's hard to resist. And sure, for some people, these medications can be effective—at least in the short term. But here's the kicker: without a solid foundation of good eating and lifestyle habits, these medications are nothing more than a temporary Band-Aid slapped over a much deeper wound. They might manage symptoms for a while, but they don't get to the root of the problem. Eventually, the benefits wear off, and guess what? The issues come creeping back, often with a few unwelcome side effects like nausea, headaches, muscle wasting, and in some cases, more serious complications like heart problems or liver damage. Not exactly the kind of trade-off you want to make, right?

So why, despite all this, do we keep going back to the diet drawing board or reaching for the next pill? As humans, we're wired to seek out quick and easy solutions with as little effort as possible. We want the magic diet that offers rapid results, lets us eat what we want, fills us up, and somehow keeps us energized, happy, and disease-free without having to lift a finger. Spoiler alert: that diet doesn't exist.

Most people don't follow their chosen diet to the letter, either. It's too restrictive, too complicated, or too time-consuming. Maybe they skip the exercise, or meal prep falls by the wayside because, let's be honest, who has the time? Sound familiar? The problem with quick-fix diets is that they're usually designed for a very specific type of person—someone who can stick to a rigid plan without any wiggle room. But here's the thing: we're all different. We have different genes, ages, stress levels, budgets, jobs, and home lives. The one-size-fits-all approach just doesn't cut it.

To truly change our eating habits and lifestyle for the better, we need to consider these individual differences. We need to understand what's making our bodies unhealthy in the first place, and then figure out the specific changes we each need to make to achieve our goals. This is where the concept of "bioindividuality" comes in—the idea that there's no one-size-fits-all approach to health and wellness. What works wonders for one person might not work at all for another. That's why most diets don't work—they don't take into account the unique needs, goals, and circumstances of each individual.

When I faced a health crisis, even as a Registered Dietitian with years of training, I turned to nutrition to heal my body. But I was just as confused as anyone else by the avalanche of conflicting advice out there. What did "turning to nutrition" even mean? I wasn't sure where to start, what to eat, or whom to trust. But despite that uncertainty, I embarked on my own health journey—and that's where the real story begins.

The Journey...

This journey began a few years ago with a diagnosis that hit me like a ton of bricks: a tumor in my eyelid that had invaded the tear ducts of my left eye. Yep, you heard that right —a tumor in my eye. Before this, I was already dealing with a laundry list of health issues: joint pain that wouldn't quit, mysterious rashes that had every doctor I saw scratching their heads, and my weight was shifting in ways I couldn't explain. And to top it all off, I just felt...crappy! I was tired, bloated, my joints ached, and my jeans? Forget about it. Suddenly, I was gaining weight—something I'd never really struggled with before (don't hate me). Oh, and did I mention I had a tumor in my eye? WAIT!!! WHAT??!!

After the eye surgeries, I thought, "Okay, maybe things will get better now." Ha! Not so fast. More skin cancers started popping up, and my health continued to spiral downward. My joint pain worsened, and my body was changing in ways that made me want to scream. After what felt like a thousand doctor visits and a mountain of tests, I finally got a diagnosis: autoimmune disease. But wait, there's more! I also found out that I had no hormone production—menopause had hit me early, before age 50. Then, as if the universe wasn't done with me yet, a large cyst developed on my ovary, leading to hemorrhaging and an emergency hysterectomy. At this point, I was practically begging the universe, *"Seriously, could it get any worse?"* My body was failing me, and I felt like I was on the losing end of a battle I didn't even know I was fighting.

As a Registered Dietitian with a master's degree in Nutritional Science, I knew deep down that food and nutrition had to be the key to my healing. But even with all my training, I was lost. Doctor after doctor handed me medications—a pill for this, a pill for that—but I knew these were just Band-Aids, temporary fixes that didn't get to the root of the problem. I needed to understand what was really going on in my body. What was the common thread pulling all these health issues together? Why was everything hitting me all at once? Determined to find answers, I dove headfirst into nutrition and holistic health literature, desperate to manage my autoimmune disease, hormone depletion, and weight gain. I even went back to school, earning an Integrative Health Coach certification from the Institute of Integrative Nutrition, with additional certifications in hormone health and gut health. I was on a mission to approach my nutrition and healing from every angle possible. Through my research, I discovered that chronic inflammation and poor gut health were the underlying culprits behind my ailments. If I was going to heal, I had to change my diet and lifestyle habits to reduce inflammation and improve gut health. Armed with this knowledge, I developed a personal protocol to kickstart my healing journey.

So, as you can see, in the beginning, it really was all about me. But as I progressed, I realized it wasn't just about me —it was about helping others who were going through similar struggles. Because if I could find a way through, so can you.

Chapter 1: Cracking The Food Code

Not long after my own health crisis, I decided to open a private nutrition counseling and coaching practice. I began working with men and women facing all sorts of chronic diseases, autoimmune disorders, and metabolic challenges. It was during this time that I had a major "light bulb" moment— one of those *Aha!* experiences where everything suddenly makes sense. I realized that, just like in my own health crisis, inflammation and poor gut health were playing leading roles in the development of many of these chronic conditions. So, naturally, if I could help my clients reduce inflammation and improve their gut health, they could see the same improvements that I did. Makes sense, right?

But here's the kicker: most people had little to no knowledge of basic nutrition or what it actually means to eat healthy. And to make matters worse, the number of people being diagnosed with chronic health conditions was skyrocketing, with many of these diagnoses happening before people even hit 40! According to the CDC, an estimated 129 million Americans have at least one chronic disease, like heart disease, cancer, diabetes, or obesity. Even more alarming, 53.8% of adults aged 18-34 already have at least one chronic condition, and 22.3% have more than one—by age 34! I mean, come on, these are the "best years" of our lives, and we're spending them dealing with health issues?

So, what's causing this? Science has shown that inflammation and gut health are often at the heart of chronic diseases and autoimmune disorders. Conditions like heart disease, diabetes, and obesity are all linked to chronic inflammation, while poor gut health can lead to issues like IBS, Crohn's disease, and other autoimmune conditions. But here's the silver lining: by eating foods that reduce inflammation and improve gut health, we can better manage and even prevent these diseases.

Now, here's another curveball: many people who desperately needed a Registered Dietitian couldn't afford one. And, honestly, dietitians in private practice (like myself) often couldn't afford to accept and manage insurance claims. So, what did people do? They turned to Dr. Google, social media influencers, or well-meaning but sometimes misguided advice from friends and family. Even worse, many healthcare practitioners would give vague directives like, "Lose 20 lbs and watch your cholesterol," without any guidance on "how" to do that. It's like giving someone a car without teaching them how to drive—no wonder people feel lost and frustrated!

And don't even get me started on the lack of nutrition education in this country. Most doctors and healthcare professionals get only a few hours to a few weeks of nutrition training in medical school. This limited exposure means they might not have the in-depth knowledge needed to provide comprehensive dietary guidance—or the time to spend with patients to offer it. As a result, patients often get inconsistent or incomplete advice about what they should be eating, leading them down the path of diet fads and misinformation.

We know that *"DIETS DON'T WORK"* because research has proven it time and time again. There's no single "diet" that can fix a chronic disease or metabolic issue. What's needed is a change in lifestyle and eating habits—personalized, tailored, and doable for each individual. These changes must be sustainable, which means they have to be understandable, practical, and affordable.

Knowing all this, I realized I needed to create a program that would teach people how to reduce inflammation through the foods they eat, while also incorporating healthier self-care and lifestyle habits. So, I took everything I had learned from my own experience and designed a program to help others RESET their metabolism by removing the foods and habits that create inflammation; REFUEL their bodies with tailored, optimal nutrition to heal their gut; and REWIRE their thinking and relationship with food, health, and self-care. Changing the way people look at their health and how they think about food, diets, and lifestyle habits seemed like a daunting task. But I was determined to create a program that would help people become the healthiest version of themselves. Because in the end, it's about more than just food—it's about cracking the code to a healthier, happier life.

The "REBOOT"

Welcome to Phil's REBOOT, a program built on the concept of bioindividuality—because let's face it, there's no one-size-fits-all when it comes to health and nutrition. We're all unique, fabulous beings, and our bodies deserve personalized habits and lifestyle changes that actually work for us long-term.

I'm beyond thrilled that you're here and that our paths have crossed! I truly hope this REBOOT program helps you achieve your optimal weight and health goals, just like it helped me. Remember, we're all works in progress, so there are three small reminders I want you to keep in mind throughout your journey:

1. **Progress Over Perfection**
2. **Be Kind To Yourself**
3. **Give Yourself Some Grace**

Just like anything worth having, this journey will require commitment and effort, but trust me—it'll be worth it! I can't wait to see all the incredible things you're going to achieve.

You Might Be Asking, "Is The REBOOT Right For Me?"

If you've been wrestling with weight loss despite trying every diet under the sun, dealing with inflammation or gut health issues, constantly feeling like you're running on empty, navigating the rollercoaster of menopause or hormonal imbalances, noticing a drop in testosterone levels, or managing conditions like heart disease, autoimmune disorders, diabetes, obesity, or even cancer—then, my friend, the REBOOT is absolutely for you!

This program is all about giving you the knowledge and tools to regain control of your health at your own pace. The REBOOT is for anyone who's tired of feeling drained, ready to reclaim their health, eager to live a more active life, or just knows it's time to make a positive change. Whatever your motivation, the REBOOT has your back with invaluable insights and support every step of the way.

Throughout our journey together, we will dive into three transformative steps:

1. **RESET**: We'll hit the reset button on your dietary habits to repair your metabolism and address (and prevent) chronic illnesses by removing inflammatory foods from your diet.

2. **REFUEL:** It's time to fuel up with wholesome, nourishing foods tailored specifically to your needs. We'll work on cultivating healthy and sustainable eating habits that fit your lifestyle.

3. **REWIRE:** Together, we'll rewire both your body and mind to optimize your metabolism and hormonal balance in a way that works for you, not against you.

The REBOOT isn't your typical diet plan. It's a comprehensive program designed to help you establish and maintain healthy dietary habits, reduce inflammation, improve gut health, manage weight and insulin levels, and create a lifestyle that helps prevent and manage chronic diseases. While there are specific guidelines to follow, there's plenty of room for personalization, ensuring the program suits *your* individual needs.

Taking on any dietary or lifestyle change requires commitment and courage, but rest assured—you're not doing this alone. We're in this together, and I promise, the rewards will be well worth the effort. Let's do this!

Breaking Down The REBOOT: What You Can Expect

The REBOOT program is like a four-course meal, each serving up something crucial for your health journey: Getting Started, RESET, REFUEL, and REWIRE. Let's dig in!

Getting Started:

In this appetizer of a chapter, we'll equip you with all the tools you need to crush the REBOOT. You'll get the lowdown on chronic inflammation, gut health, and how these sneaky culprits mess with your weight, digestion, immunity, and hormones. Chronic inflammation is no joke—it's linked to all sorts of nasties like heart disease, diabetes, and autoimmune disorders. Plus, you'll learn how gut health is the unsung hero of your overall well-being, affecting everything from digestion to mood. By the end of this chapter, you'll be armed with knowledge and strategies to give those health woes the boot.

RESET:

Now, onto the main course—think of this as your personal "elimination" challenge. During RESET, you'll gradually cut out inflammatory foods from your diet. Don't worry, we'll guide you through it step by step, giving you a list of foods to embrace and those to avoid like the plague.

This phase is all about hitting the reset button on your gut and metabolism by detoxing from inflammation-triggering foods and toxins. As you progress, expect to feel the benefits rolling in—less inflammation, better digestion, more energy, and a metabolism that's ready to work "with" you, not against you.

REFUEL:

Now that you've cleared the clutter, it's time to restock the pantry with the good stuff. In the REFUEL phase, you'll learn how to reintroduce foods strategically, supporting decreased inflammation and improved gut health. We'll help you swap out the bad guys for healthier alternatives, giving you a personalized eating plan that's as delicious as it is nutritious.

By the end of REFUEL, you'll have a solid understanding of how different foods affect your body and a customized plan that keeps you feeling your best. This phase is all about taking control of your health one tasty meal at a time.

REWIRE:

Finally, we serve up dessert with a side of self-care. By this point, you've transformed your relationship with food and your mindset around nutrition. In REWIRE, we'll help you lock in those changes and keep evolving towards a healthier body and mind.

Self-care isn't just a buzzword—it's the glue that holds your progress together. We'll show you how to incorporate habits that support both your physical and mental health, from nourishing meals to stress-busting practices.

As you work through REWIRE, you'll gain a deeper appreciation for how these self-care practices contribute to your overall happiness and well-being. And because the REBOOT is all about you, you can customize the program to fit your life.

The Flexibility of the REBOOT

The magic of the REBOOT lies in its flexibility and adaptability to your individual needs. We've loaded you up with a variety of tools and resources, allowing you to tailor the program to fit your lifestyle. Want to dive deep and use every single resource? Go for it! Prefer to pick and choose what works best for you? That's perfectly fine, too.

We offer access to a private Facebook group, comprehensive grocery lists, mouthwatering recipes, handy snack suggestions, pantry essentials, and more tools to help you track progress and stay accountable. The best part? You can use as much or as little of these resources as you like, based on your needs, learning style, and preferences. Whether you engage fully with the program or select specific components that suit your journey, the REBOOT is here to support you every step of the way.

Prelude To Chapter Two: Setting The Stage

Before we dive into Chapter Two, let's take a moment to acknowledge where we're headed. We've already talked about why diets don't work and shared some of the struggles that brought us here. Now, it's time to arm ourselves with the knowledge that will set us up for success on this journey.

In Chapter Two, we're going to cover the basics—the essential nutrition information that's often overlooked or misunderstood. Think of this chapter as your backstage pass to understanding what's really going on with your body and your food. You'll learn about the building blocks of good health, the truth behind common food myths, and the key principles that will guide you through the REBOOT.

Expect some lightbulb moments, a few "Aha!" realizations, and maybe even a couple of chuckles as we break down these concepts in a way that's easy to understand and (dare I say) even enjoyable. By the end of this chapter, you'll be equipped with the foundational knowledge you need to navigate the rest of the REBOOT with confidence. So, get ready to dive in—this is where the real fun begins!

Now, let's get started!

Chapter 2: Basic Nutrition 101

Let's be honest: most Americans get about as much nutrition education as they get training in rocket science—yet health professionals love to tell them to lose weight, lower their cholesterol, or manage their blood sugar as if it's the easiest thing in the world. The problem? They often don't get the "how" to go with the "what". This lack of guidance sends people down the rabbit hole of the internet, where they search for nutrition advice and end up drowning in a sea of misinformation, confusion, and, let's face it, a little bit of despair.

Without the right knowledge or support, people end up following questionable advice, struggling to reach their health goals, and feeling completely overwhelmed by all the conflicting information out there. That's why, before we dive into the "REBOOT," I want to clear up some key nutrition concepts. We'll make sure you know the difference between things like inflammation and gut health so you've got a solid foundation to build on as you embark on your journey to better health. Consider this your pre-REBOOT pep talk—let's get you ready to tackle those health goals with confidence!

Let's Talk About INFLAMMATION...

Alright, let's start with the basics: inflammation. Is it good or bad? Well, the answer is both!

Acute inflammation is actually your body's way of helping you out. Think of it as the first responder when you cut your finger. Your body sends out inflammatory cells to the rescue, starting the healing process. This kind of inflammation is your body doing its job and usually clears up in a few days.

Chronic inflammation, though, is a different story—and not a good one. Imagine those first responders never leaving the scene and instead setting up camp for weeks, months, or even years. Chronic inflammation sticks around too long, quietly wreaking havoc on your health without you even realizing it. It often flies under the radar because it doesn't cause the obvious pain or discomfort that acute inflammation does. But the symptoms are there, lurking in the form of fatigue, brain fog, joint pain, weight gain, and even depression.

Chronic inflammation has been linked to a laundry list of diseases, including obesity, diabetes, heart disease, arthritis, and even Alzheimer's. And here's the kicker: it's not just an "old person" problem. More and more young people are dealing with chronic inflammation, leading to poor health and a lower quality of life much earlier than you'd expect.

For women, inflammation is especially tricky around menopause. Hormonal changes can start as early as your late 30s and can last 2-8 years (yes, you read that right—years!). During this time, you might notice more sugar cravings, weight gain around your middle, sleep issues, and mood swings—all of which fuel a vicious cycle of inflammation and hormone imbalance.

Gentlemen, don't think you're off the hook. Inflammation doesn't discriminate, and it can lead to heart disease, cancer, and diabetes in men too. But the good news for everyone is that with the right nutrition, you can fight back.

And let's not forget about **"INFLAMMAGING"**—a term that describes the chronic, low-grade inflammation that speeds up the aging process. This isn't just about wrinkles and gray hair; it's about the way inflammation contributes to age-related diseases like heart disease and Alzheimer's. But there's hope! By addressing inflammation through diet, exercise, and stress management, you can slow down the aging process and improve your overall health. So, while we can't stop getting older, we can certainly try to age gracefully by kicking chronic inflammation to the curb!

Let's Talk About the Food-Inflammation Connection

Alright, here's the scoop: what you eat has a direct impact on the bacteria in your gut and the chemicals they produce during digestion. These chemicals can either fan the flames of inflammation or help put them out.

Take sugar, for example—especially the sneaky kind hiding in high fructose corn syrup, along with refined carbs like white bread, cookies, and cakes. These culprits can lead to insulin resistance, diabetes, and obesity. It's like sending an open invitation for inflammation to crash your party. Studies have also shown that munching on processed and packaged foods loaded with trans fats can damage the cells lining your blood vessels, paving the way for heart disease. And let's not forget about alcohol and processed meats—overdoing it on these can spark some serious inflammation.

On the flip side, there's good news: an anti-inflammatory diet can help lower these risks. While there are plenty of "anti-inflammatory" diets out there, they all boil down to a few basic principles that should be the foundation of your eating plan. We'll dive into these principles as we go through

26

the book and embrace the REBOOT. In short, think of your diet as the fire extinguisher for inflammation—choose wisely, and you'll keep those flames under control!

Gut Health & The Immune System: Prebiotics, Probiotics, and Fiber

Let's dive into gut health, the buzzword of the decade! If you haven't heard of gut health or the gut microbiome, no worries—I've got you covered. Gut health is all about having a happy digestive system, free from annoying issues like gas, bloating, and diarrhea, and avoiding conditions like leaky gut and inflammation of the gut lining.

Your gut is home to a bustling community of microorganisms—think of it as a tiny city living inside you. This community is known as your gut flora, gut microbiota, or gut microbiome, and it's made up of around 100 trillion bacteria (both good and bad) that collectively weigh about 5 pounds! These little guys are crucial because they influence almost every organ in your body and play a huge role in your metabolism.

Your gut is basically the body's nutritional hub. It breaks down food, absorbs nutrients, and converts them into energy. To keep your overall health in check, it's super important to keep your gut in balance, making sure the good bacteria outnumber the bad ones.

Most of your gut flora hangs out in your large intestine (aka the colon), which is the final stop in your digestive tract. Here, they work their magic by making vitamins like vitamin K and some B vitamins, and by converting fibers into short-chain fatty acids such as butyrate, propionate, and acetate. These fatty acids are like super fuel for your gut wall, help with metabolism, boost your immune system, and keep your gut wall strong to prevent unwanted stuff from sneaking into your body.

The tricky part? Your gut flora is super sensitive to what you eat. Poor gut health is linked to a whole list of issues, like obesity, type 2 diabetes, heart disease, colorectal cancer, Alzheimer's, and even depression. But don't worry—having a variety of bacteria in your gut can help reduce the risk of these conditions.

Research shows that 70-80% of your immune cells are chilling in your gut, making it the largest immune organ in your body. This means your gut health and immune system are BFFs. There's even a strong connection between your gut and brain, known as the gut-brain axis. This connection can affect your mood, behavior, and mental health, linking gut health to conditions like anxiety and depression.

The gut and brain are connected by the "vagus nerve," which runs from your brain to your colon. This nerve helps regulate digestion, appetite, and even vitamin B12 uptake. A healthy vagus nerve can keep things moving (literally), and help you absorb nutrients like a pro.

When there's inflammation in your gut (think too many bad bacteria), it can mess with your mental and emotional well-being, potentially leading to depression. Your gut also produces and stores hormones and neurotransmitters. Fun fact: about 90% of your serotonin—the feel-good hormone—is produced in your gut. So, a happy gut means a happy you!

How the Brain Influences the Gut:

Let's talk about the brain-gut connection—because, yes, your brain and gut are in constant communication, and they have quite the relationship! When you're exposed to prolonged or chronic stress, your vagus nerve (the nerve that connects your brain to your gut) can start acting up. This can lead to stalled digestion and all sorts of gut issues that nobody asked for. It's like your brain is throwing a wrench into your digestive system.

Now, let's not forget how important diet is in this equation. What you eat directly impacts your gut microbiota and your immune system. If your gut isn't in tip-top shape, neither your immune nor digestive systems will function properly. It's really that simple! But many things can throw your gut out of whack—stress, lack of sleep, a diet full of processed and sugary foods, alcohol, and the overuse of antibiotics.

Symptoms of Poor Gut Health Include:
- Upset stomach
- Gastrointestinal distress
- Unintentional weight changes
- Small intestine bacterial overgrowth (SIBO)
- Sleep disturbances
- Fatigue
- Skin conditions like psoriasis
- Autoimmune conditions
- Food intolerances

Research shows that the best way to keep your gut happy is to limit antibiotics, NSAIDS, and alcohol, and focus on a nutrient-dense, mostly plant-based diet rich in fermented and whole foods, and high in fiber. Unfortunately, the typical Western diet (aka the Standard American Diet, or SAD) is loaded with sugars and processed foods that can damage your gut lining, leading to inflammation and a whole host of health issues.

So, what's the takeaway? Feed your gut well with plenty of prebiotics, probiotics, and fiber, and it will pay you back with good health and a smoother digestive journey. Think of it as your gut's way of saying, "Thanks for the good eats!"

What Are PRE-biotics?

So, what's the deal with prebiotics? Think of them as the snacks for the good bacteria in your gut. Prebiotics are non-digestible food ingredients that serve as nourishment for the beneficial bacteria already living in your digestive system. These little helpers, like certain types of fiber, aren't digested by your body. Instead, they head straight to your gut to feed the good bacteria, helping them thrive and do their job better.

When you consume prebiotics, you're essentially fueling the production of nutrients that benefit your colon cells, leading to a healthier digestive system overall. And here's the bonus: prebiotics don't just feed your gut bacteria; they also have anti-inflammatory effects and boost the absorption of important minerals like calcium and magnesium. So, in a way, prebiotics are like the ultimate multi-taskers for your gut health —feeding the good guys while keeping the bad stuff in check!

Prebiotic Foods for a Healthy Gut Microbiome:

- Chicory Root
- Dandelion Greens
- Jerusalem Artichoke
- Onions
- Garlic
- Leeks
- Asparagus
- Bananas
- Barley
- Oats
- Apples
- Konjac Root
- Burdock Root
- Jicama Root
- Avocado
- Cocoa
- Flaxseed
- Wheat Bran
- Seaweed

What Are PRO-biotics?

Probiotics are like the VIP guests in the gut health party —they're the live microorganisms (mostly bacteria) that, when consumed, bring some serious health benefits to the table. According to the National Center for Complementary and Integrative Health, probiotics can strengthen your gut, aid digestion, and keep everything in balance. When your gut gets out of whack (think more bad bacteria than good), probiotics step in to restore order.

But that's not all—these tiny powerhouses may also help with weight loss, digestion, neurological disorders, heart health, immune function, and even symptoms of depression and anxiety. Researchers are pouring billions into studying the human microbiome, and they're just scratching the surface of what probiotics can do!

It's important to note that not all probiotics are created equal; different types have different effects on your body. And the good news? You can find probiotics in many foods, so you can easily invite these gut-friendly guests into your diet.

Probiotic-Rich Foods:

- Yogurt (with live cultures)
- Kefir
- Sauerkraut
- Kimchi
- Miso
- Tempeh
- Kombucha
- Traditional Buttermilk
- Natto
- Pickles and Pickled Vegetables
- Cheeses with live/active cultures, such as:
  - Cheddar
  - Mozzarella

How To Choose a Probiotic

So, you're thinking about adding a probiotic to your routine—great idea! But here's the thing: getting enough probiotics "naturally" through food can be tricky, so you might need to reach for a supplement. But before you do, keep in mind that probiotics aren't a one-size-fits-all deal. They might not be suitable for everyone, especially if you're undergoing chemotherapy or dealing with conditions like Crohn's disease, histamine intolerance, IBS, SIBO, IBD, or ulcerative colitis. If you're unsure whether a probiotic supplement is right for you, it's always a good idea to chat with a Registered Dietitian or your healthcare provider first.

Now, here's the kicker—probiotics are considered dietary supplements, not drugs, so they're not regulated by the FDA. That means it's up to you to do your homework before picking one. Lucky for you, there's a great article out there that breaks down the top-rated probiotic supplements (as recommended by dietitians) and how to choose the right one for your needs. Just remember, as with any new supplement or medication, it's always safer to get the thumbs up from your healthcare provider before diving in. So, go ahead, get those gut-friendly bacteria on board—just make sure you're choosing the right team! Article: https://www.healthline.com/nutrition/best-probiotic-supplement

Dietary Fiber

Let's talk fiber—nature's broom for your gut! Dietary fiber is the part of plant cells that your body's enzymes just can't break down. Instead of getting digested, fiber passes through your stomach untouched and heads straight to your colon, where it becomes a feast for your "good" gut bacteria—also known as prebiotics.

According to The American Heart Association, fiber does more than just keep things moving. It's been shown to protect against heart disease, diabetes, inflammatory bowel disease, obesity, and even colorectal cancer. Plus, fiber helps flush out toxins, lowers cholesterol, and can even help you shed some pounds by keeping you fuller for longer with fewer calories. Much of these benefits are thanks to your gut microbiota. See how it's all connected?

Fiber is technically a carbohydrate, but unlike most carbs, your body can't break it down, so it passes through undigested. But not all fiber is created equal—there are two types: soluble and insoluble.

Soluble fiber dissolves in water and acts like a superhero for your gut, providing food for the good bacteria. Think of it as the guest of honor at the gut bacteria banquet.

Insoluble fiber, on the other hand, doesn't dissolve in water and isn't as popular with the bacteria, but it's still important for keeping things moving along smoothly in your digestive tract. So, when you're loading up on fiber, remember you're not just doing it for you—you're feeding the good guys in your gut too!

Soluble Fiber:
- Barley
- Oatmeal
- Beans
- Nuts
- Fruits such as apples, berries, citrus fruits, and

Insoluble Fiber:
- Whole grains
- Wheat cereals
- Vegetables such as carrots, celery, and tomatoes

The American Heart Association suggests aiming for 25-30 grams of dietary fiber per day. While it's best to meet this goal through nutrient-dense, whole foods, let's be real—it's not always easy to pack that much fiber into your meals. That's where a fiber supplement might come in handy. But here's a pro tip: don't dive headfirst into high-fiber territory! Gradually increase your intake to avoid any unwanted side effects like bloating and gas. Your digestive system will thank you for easing into it, and you'll still reap all those wonderful fiber benefits!

Water and Hydration: What's the Big Deal?

Let's talk about water—because it's kind of a big deal. In fact, water makes up about 60% of your body weight and 90% of your blood. It's essential for keeping everything in your body running smoothly and, you know, keeping you alive! Without water, most of us wouldn't last more than three days. So yeah, it's pretty important!

Water does more than just quench your thirst. It plays a ton of vital roles in your body, including helping with weight loss. Some studies suggest that drinking water can make you feel fuller (yay, less snacking!) and even give your metabolism a little boost. And if you swap out sugary drinks for good ol H2O, you'll not only cut calories but also reduce inflammation and avoid weight gain. But weight loss is just one of water's many superpowers.

Here's a quick rundown of what water does for you: It boosts physical performance, keeping you strong during workouts, and supports your energy levels and brain function, helping to prevent fatigue and brain fog. Staying hydrated can fend off headaches and relieve constipation by keeping things moving smoothly in your digestive system. After a night out, water becomes your best friend in preventing hangovers, and it also helps treat kidney stones by flushing them out. Water plays a crucial role in regulating body temperature, keeping you cool in the heat and warm in the cold. It moistens tissues, keeping your eyes, nose, and mouth hydrated, and creates saliva, which is vital for tasting and digesting food. Water also protects your organs and tissues by acting as a cushion and carries nutrients and oxygen to your cells. It lubricates your joints for smooth movement and helps your body flush out waste and toxins. Additionally, water dissolves nutrients and minerals, making them easier for your body to absorb.

So, the next time you're thinking about what your body needs to stay healthy, remember: water is a big deal. Keep that bottle handy, and your body will thank you! After all, if your body is like a well-oiled machine, then water is the oil that keeps all those gears running smoothly—so don't let yourself run dry!

How Much Water Do You Need?

Wondering how much water you should be guzzling each day? The National Academy of Medicine recommends about 13 cups (104 ounces) for healthy men and 9 cups (72 ounces) for healthy women. Keep in mind, one cup equals 8 ounces. If you're hitting the gym hard or spending time in a hot climate, you might need to up your intake. On the flip side, if you're on the smaller side, you might not need as much. But remember, this isn't a strict daily target—more of a ballpark figure.

Here's a little tip: if you're feeling thirsty, your body is already a bit dehydrated.

Dehydration isn't just about feeling parched—it can actually stir up inflammation in your body. When you're not getting enough water, your body struggles to detoxify, leading to a buildup of toxins and waste that can trigger inflammation. Dehydration also decreases blood volume and lymphatic fluids, making it tougher for your immune cells to do their job. Plus, it hampers the delivery of oxygen and nutrients to your cells, meaning your body doesn't function as well as it should. So, staying hydrated is key to keeping everything running smoothly and keeping inflammation at bay!

Some signs that you might be dehydrated include headaches or confusion, tiredness and fatigue, dizziness, weakness, or feeling light-headed. You might notice a dry mouth or even a dry cough, and your heart rate could be high while your blood pressure drops. Dehydration can also make you lose your appetite (though you might start craving sugar), and you might feel flushed, get swollen feet, experience muscle cramps, or even develop heat intolerance or chills. Constipation is another telltale sign, and if your urine is dark-colored instead of a pale lemonade shade, it's time to drink up!

So, keep that water bottle close—your body will thank you! Think of it as your hydration sidekick, always there to save the day and keep your body in superhero shape!

Ways to Stay Hydrated

Staying hydrated can feel like a chore, especially if you're not naturally inclined to reach for that water bottle. But don't worry, I've got a few tips to make it a little easier—and maybe even a little fun!

Start your day like a hydration pro: before you even think about your morning coffee, gulp down a tall glass of water. It's like giving your body a refreshing wake-up call! Throughout the day, keep a water container by your side as your trusty companion. And why not make a game out of it? Set daily water goals and challenge yourself to hit them—no cheating!

If plain water doesn't do it for you, no problem! Jazz it up with a slice of organic lemon or lime, or toss in some mint, basil leaves, or fresh/frozen organic fruit. Think of it as turning your water into a mini spa experience—who wouldn't want to sip on that all day?

Electrolyte Supplementation:

The health food market is flooded with "electrolyte supplements" these days, all claiming to help with dehydration. But before you start grabbing them off the shelf, let's break down what electrolytes actually are, where to find them naturally, and how to pick a good supplement if you need one.

Electrolytes are essential minerals like sodium, potassium, chloride, calcium, magnesium, phosphate, and bicarbonate. These little powerhouses are crucial for keeping your body in balance, ensuring your nerves and muscles work properly, and keeping you hydrated. The good news is, if you eat a well-balanced diet full of nutritious foods and drinks, you're probably getting most of the electrolytes you need.

Load up on fruits and vegetables rich in electrolytes, and don't forget other healthy sources like avocados, berries, dairy products, certain grains, and seafood like salmon and shellfish. And, of course, stay hydrated throughout the day—your body will thank you!

If you're someone who exercises regularly, it's important to pay attention to your fluid intake. For those mild to moderate workouts, plain old water usually does the trick. But if you're really pushing yourself or exercising for a long stretch, you might want to consider adding an electrolyte drink into the mix. The same goes if you're dealing with less-than-pleasant situations like diarrhea or vomiting—keeping an oral electrolyte solution handy, like coconut water, can be a lifesaver to prevent dehydration.

Now, when choosing an electrolyte supplement, keep a few things in mind. First off, skip the sugar! Look for options with little to no added sugars; monk fruit is a great alternative. Avoid anything with artificial additives—keep it clean and natural. Always check the ingredients list for natural sources, and remember, more isn't always better, so watch that serving size! It's also worth picking a reputable brand—quality matters, so do a little research. Reading reviews can give you a good idea of what others think, and look for supplements that have undergone third-party testing to ensure they meet high standards. Finally, make sure the supplement fits your dietary needs, whether that's gluten-free, vegan, or otherwise.

If you've been feeling a bit dehydrated and decide to supplement with natural foods or a carefully chosen electrolyte drink, you should start to feel better. But if your symptoms persist, it might be time to have a chat with your healthcare provider. Stay hydrated, stay healthy, and remember—when it comes to electrolytes, more isn't always better!

Sources Of Water

There has been a lot of research done on the safety of your drinking water, as well as the "best kind" of water to drink. Use the link below to the Environmental Working Group's (WEG) "Guide To Safe Drinking Water," as well as EWG's "Water Filter Guide." If you're not familiar with the EWG, it is a nonprofit, nonpartisan organization dedicated to helping you live your healthiest life. There are many great resources on their website! https://www.ewg.org, and they can always use your support to continue doing amazing work!

Intermittent Fasting 101

So, you've probably heard the buzz about intermittent fasting (IF), right? It's all the rage in diet circles, and some plans even make it a requirement. But here's the deal: IF is totally OPTIONAL during your REBOOT journey. You can try it out anytime—or not at all. No pressure!

What Is Intermittent Fasting (IF)?

Intermittent Fasting is basically a fancy way of saying you cycle between periods of eating and not eating. Think of it as giving your digestive system a little vacation between meals.

Who Should Skip Intermittent Fasting?

IF isn't for everyone. If you're under 18 or over 75, dealing with fertility issues, pregnant or breastfeeding, managing diabetes, on certain meds, a hardcore endurance athlete, have a history of disordered eating, or have specific medical conditions like kidney disease—IF might not be your jam. When in doubt, always check with a healthcare professional before diving in.

Which Fasting Plan Should You Choose?

Pick the fasting plan that fits your lifestyle. There are several options, like the 20:4 Plan, the 16:8 Plan, the 5:2 Fasting Plan, and the Alternate Day Fasting Plan. For our purposes, we'll focus on the 16:8 Plan.

What Does a 16:8 Plan Actually Mean?

The 16:8 method of intermittent fasting is a popular approach that involves fasting for 16 hours each day and restricting your eating window to the remaining 8 hours. For example, if you choose to eat between 12:00 PM and 8:00 PM, you would fast from 8:00 PM until 12:00 PM the next day. During the 16-hour fasting period, only non-caloric beverages like water, tea, or black coffee are typically consumed. This method is favored by many because it easily fits into a daily routine, allowing for flexibility in food choices while still providing the benefits of intermittent fasting, such as improved metabolic health and weight management. The idea is to give your body an extended break from digestion, which can promote fat burning, improve insulin sensitivity, and potentially support longevity.

We're going with a "clean fast" approach here, meaning nothing with calories during your fasting period. You can repeat this cycle as often as you like—whether that's a few times a week or every day, it's up to you. The 16:8 plan tends to offer the best balance of satisfaction, stable energy levels, and mood.

Taking Medications and Supplements During IF:

If you need to take meds with food or have specific timing requirements, IF might not be for you. Also, if you take supplements that are better absorbed with food (like vitamins A, D, E, K), save those for your first meal of the day. Most other vitamins won't break your fast, so you're good to go with those.

What Does IF Do to Your Body?

When you fast, some pretty cool things happen inside your body. Your hormone levels adjust to make fat more available for energy, and your cells kick into repair mode, including some genetic tweaking while you sleep.

Health Benefits of IF:

Intermittent fasting (IF) comes with a host of health benefits that make it more than just a trendy buzzword. First up, it increases Human Growth Hormone (HGH), which not only helps with fat loss but also boosts muscle gain—think of it as a two-for-one deal for your body. It also improves insulin sensitivity, making fat more accessible as an energy source, which is great news for those targeting stubborn belly fat.

But that's not all. IF reduces oxidative stress and inflammation, lowering your risk of chronic diseases, and it may even offer some protection against Alzheimer's disease by slowing its effects. Thanks to a process called autophagy, your cells also get a chance to "clean house," removing old, dysfunctional proteins that can clog up your system. Lowering inflammation markers and LDL "bad" cholesterol, IF also contributes to overall better health and reduces heart disease risk. Improved gene function supports longevity and disease protection, making IF a potential key to living longer.

However, a quick reality check: even with all these benefits, what you eat during your eating window still matters. Quality and quantity are crucial to your success and overall health. So remember, you really are what you eat—so make those choices count!

What to Eat When Intermittent Fasting

When you're diving into intermittent fasting, it's all about fueling your body with the good stuff during your eating windows. Think whole, nutrient-dense foods and full-fat goodies. Foods like avocados, nuts, seeds, and dairy (hold off on the dairy during the RESET—we'll get to that later) are your best friends here. These full-fat options not only keep you feeling full but also provide essential fatty acids and fat-soluble vitamins that your body loves. Plus, they help you avoid that hangry feeling and make sticking to your fasting schedule a breeze.

The steady energy you get from healthy fats can also help you avoid the dreaded blood sugar rollercoaster that comes with high-carb snacks. Just remember, even though these fats are good for you, moderation is key—nobody wants to end up eating more calories than they burn!

What to Eat When Breaking Your Fast

When it's time to break your fast, you'll want to give your body the good stuff. Focus on nutrient-packed foods that help balance your blood sugar and keep you feeling satisfied. Think of it as refueling your body with a mix of lean protein (like chicken, fish, or organic tofu), healthy fats (like avocados, nuts, or olive oil), and complex carbs (whole grains, veggies, or fruits). Adding fiber-rich foods is also a great idea—they'll keep your digestion running smoothly and help you stay full longer.

Bone broth is another superstar for breaking your fast. It's easy on the stomach and loaded with nutrients. Just be sure to skip the high-sugar or processed foods—they might seem tempting, but they can spike your blood sugar and undo some of the benefits of your fasting efforts.

Are Keto and Intermittent Fasting the Same Thing?

Not at all! While intermittent fasting (IF) is all about *when* you eat, the Keto diet focuses on "what" and "how much" you eat. Before you jump into Keto, let's talk about the risks...

Sure, Keto might seem like the magic solution for weight loss, but it can have some pretty serious side effects if followed long-term. First, you might run into nutrient deficiencies because cutting out certain food groups means missing out on key vitamins and minerals. Then there's the infamous "Keto Flu," where you might experience headaches, fatigue, and nausea as your body adapts to low carbs—fun, right?

But the fun doesn't stop there. Low fiber intake on Keto can lead to some, shall we say, less-than-pleasant digestive issues like constipation. And while you're loading up on those high saturated fats, keep in mind they can raise your bad cholesterol (LDL) levels, increasing your heart disease risk. Keto also ups your chances of developing kidney stones and puts extra strain on your liver as it works overtime to metabolize all that fat. Not to mention, there's potential for decreased bone density, which could raise your risk of fractures.

If that's not enough, there's the risk of hypoglycemia (especially for diabetics) and reduced athletic performance—because who doesn't want to feel sluggish during a workout? Oh, and let's not forget about sustainability. Keto can be tough to stick with long-term, and it might even lead to social isolation because, let's face it, how many social gatherings are carb-free?

Before diving into the deep end of the Keto pool, it's always a good idea to check with a healthcare professional, especially if you have any preexisting health conditions. After all, your health is worth more than a quick-fix diet trend!

Intermittent fasting is generally a healthier and more sustainable option, especially when combined with the REBOOT. The REBOOT is designed to help you create healthier eating habits by focusing on whole foods like grains, legumes, nuts, organic fruits and veggies, lean meats, pastured eggs, and wild-caught seafood. These foods are known to reduce inflammation and chronic disease.

You can start intermittent fasting anytime during the REBOOT, or skip it altogether if it doesn't feel right for you. This is your journey, and it's important to set yourself up for success. Remember, it took years to develop your current habits, so it'll take time to create healthier ones.

Give yourself some grace—you're making progress, and that's what counts!

Women and Fasting

Alright, ladies, let's talk about the good, the bad, and the hormonal when it comes to intermittent fasting. According to the Cleveland Clinic, women can absolutely benefit from intermittent fasting, just like men. We're talking weight loss, better immunity, reduced inflammation, regulated blood sugar, improved gut health, decreased appetite, better blood pressure, and lower triglycerides. Sounds great, right? But here's the kicker: intermittent fasting can mess with those all-important female hormones—progesterone and estrogen. And because of these hormones, the results for women often aren't as dramatic as they are for men. I know, totally unfair, right?

Hormone levels in women are like a rollercoaster, rising and falling throughout the menstrual cycle. When these hormones peak, it's ovulation time—the prime window for pregnancy. But intermittent fasting can confuse your body, sending signals that food is scarce and potentially causing your menstrual cycle to go haywire. We're talking skipped periods, mood swings, low sex drive, dry skin, hair loss, acne, disrupted sleep, heart palpitations, and even infertility. Not exactly what we signed up for!

If you're still menstruating, here are a few tips:

Try shortening your fasting times during the two weeks leading up to your period. Trust me, your body will thank you. Also, it's wise to avoid fasting altogether in the week before your period. Your body is more sensitive to stress during this time, and the drop in estrogen doesn't make things any easier. And here's an important note—if you're pregnant, breastfeeding, or trying to conceive, intermittent fasting is a no-go. Always check with your healthcare provider before making any big changes.

The key takeaway? Listen to your body! Every woman's hormonal needs and overall health are unique, so it's crucial to tailor your fasting approach accordingly. Now, for the postmenopausal women out there, the story is a bit different. Since you're not dealing with the same hormone fluctuations, intermittent fasting might actually be more beneficial in your 50s, 60s, and beyond. However, if you're still experiencing low hormone symptoms after menopause, it's always a good idea to consult with a healthcare provider to make sure intermittent fasting is the right fit for you.

Congratulations! You've now got all the tools and knowledge you need to tackle the REBOOT with clarity and confidence.

We have covered everything from the basics of nutrition to the nitty-gritty details of how your body reacts to different foods and habits. Whether it's understanding the impact of inflammation, navigating the world of gut health, or mastering intermittent fasting, you're fully equipped to make informed choices that support your health goals. So go ahead, dive into the REBOOT, and trust that you've got this—you're ready to take on this journey with all the confidence in the world!

Chapter 3: Getting Started

Alright, REBOOTERS, before we dive headfirst into Cracking The Food Code and setting you on the path to creating the healthiest version of yourself, we've got a little prep work to handle—think of it as setting the stage for your success. Just like you wouldn't start cooking without first gathering all your ingredients, we need to tackle some essential housekeeping tasks to get you fully prepped and ready to crush this journey.

These steps aren't just busywork; they're designed to help you glide through the REBOOT with less stress and more confidence. So, grab your metaphorical mop, because we're about to tidy up, get organized, and set you up for a win. And don't worry—I'll be here to keep things light and fun as we get everything in order! Ready to crack the code? Let's do this!

1. *Get Ready, Get Set, Almost There...I Need To Find My REBOOT Mojo! The Power of Mindset*

When I embarked on this journey, I found myself in a state of physical and emotional turmoil, facing one health setback after another. It felt like I was caught in a never-ending loop of failed diet attempts and mounting frustration—a place I'm sure many of you have been. I was disheartened, defeated, and overwhelmed by the challenges before me. It was during this pivotal moment that I realized the importance of cultivating the right mindset to confront my circumstances head-on. So, I called Kim Johnson, my dear friend and trusted mindset coach.

Kim has been immersed in the world of self-development since 1996, learning from leading professionals, including Tony Robbins, with whom she spent nearly 18 years. Initially, Kim's journey into self-development was driven by her desire to improve her personal and professional life. Little did she know, it would become her true calling. While she explored various ventures—from owning an ad agency to running a gelato shop—Kim's true passion lay in teaching, writing, and coaching. This passion has led her to accumulate over 45,000 coaching hours, touch the lives of thousands, author eight books (including two bestsellers), host a daily podcast, and create a fulfilling life surrounded by her family, numerous animals, and a lively chicken coop.

Kim's invaluable contributions have been instrumental in shaping the REBOOT and guiding me on my journey of self-discovery and growth. Through her mentorship, I've learned to cultivate the mindset necessary to pursue my goals and determine the version of myself I choose to embody each day. Kim has a unique gift for asking the tough, probing questions that dig deep into your psyche, and while that can be daunting, it's also incredibly rewarding. I am deeply grateful for Kim—for her wisdom, unwavering support, and cherished friendship.

If you're seeking to harness control over your emotions and cultivate a winning mindset, I wholeheartedly recommend reading Kim's book, "Who's Driving Your Bus?", available on Amazon. It's a transformative read that offers profound insights into the power of mindset and personal growth.

Now, let me hand it over to Kim, who's going to share some insights that are crucial as you embark on this journey with me. Trust me, her advice is pure gold, and I'm beyond excited that she's a part of this book to guide you through the mindset shifts that are just as important as the nutrition changes we're going to make. So, without further ado, here's Kim to help you get your mind in the right place as we start this REBOOT together!

A Message From Kim...

Hey everybody, I'm Kim Johnson, and I am thrilled to be part of this book with Phil. I'm here to help you understand your mindset as you embark on the REBOOT. You're in for a treat with Phil's incredible insights and training, which will completely transform your relationship with food.

My focus is on mindset. As you progress through this program, the most important thing I can share is that while you'll gain valuable tools, success hinges on your mindset. If you're not mentally prepared, these tools won't be as effective. You need to shift your identity, your patterns, and your thinking. Essentially, the distance between you and success is measured by how far you can stretch your mind.

Throughout the REBOOT, remember to ask yourself the right questions. If you find yourself struggling and asking, "Why is this so hard?" it's those questions that are holding you back. You must change your thought process and your questions to align with a success-oriented mindset.

Visualize the version of yourself you'll be at the end of this course. Whether it's the 2.0, 3.0, or 4.0 version, that better version of you should be in control of your mindset during the REBOOT.

I wrote a book called "Who's Driving Your Bus?" which focuses on controlling your mindset. This book will help you understand your mind chatter, enhance your success, and provide you with the tools to stay on the right path. If you ever feel stuck, the best thing you can do is reach out for help. Acknowledging that you need assistance opens you up to new possibilities. Staying silent and isolated won't benefit you.

Pay attention to your inner dialogue and change how you communicate with yourself. I promise, the results will be amazing once you do.

Good luck, enjoy the book, and have fun with Phil and the REBOOT!

2. *Get Ready, Get Set, Almost There…Wait, Did I Take My "Before" Photo?…Tracking Your Progress*

As you kick off your REBOOT journey, tracking your progress can be a game-changer. It's like having a map for your personal transformation—letting you see where you started, how far you've come, and where you're headed. Plus, who doesn't love celebrating those small victories along the way? Here are a few tips to get you started:

A. Weigh Yourself: Start by hopping on the scale before you dive into the REBOOT. Jot down your starting weight, but remember, this is just one piece of the puzzle—don't let it define your success!

B. Baseline Blood Work: If you're really serious about seeing the changes, consider getting some baseline blood work done. It'll give you a clear snapshot of your starting point, so you can watch those numbers improve as you go.

C. Before Photo: Snap a "before" photo—you'll thank yourself later when you can look back and see just how far you've come. Plus, it's great motivation to keep pushing forward!

These little check-ins aren't about being hard on yourself; they're about celebrating every win, no matter how small. So, track your progress, and let those milestones remind you of just how awesome you're doing on this journey to better health!

3. Get Ready, Get Set, Almost There...Let Me Just Cultivate a Bit More Gratitude!

As you embark on this journey, documenting your progress is a powerful tool. Take time to record your measurements and personal reflections in a journal—it's your private space to track your journey, capture your thoughts, and preserve the experiences you'll have throughout this program. Putting pen to paper might seem simple, but it's one of the most effective tools for wellness. Your journal isn't just for tracking numbers; it can also be a vessel for practicing gratitude—a transformative habit that shifts your focus to the positive aspects of your life.

Gratitude is a conscious choice, and like any habit, it grows stronger with practice. At first, it might feel a bit awkward or forced, but over time, it becomes second nature. Research shows that cultivating gratitude can activate your parasympathetic nervous system—your body's "rest and digest" response. In other words, practicing gratitude can significantly boost positivity and contribute to overall happiness.

But let's be real... some days, finding things to be grateful for might feel like trying to find a needle in a haystack. That's okay—it happens to the best of us. This is where I come in. I often ask my clients what they're grateful for, and sometimes, I get silence. They look at me like, "Really, Phil? Today?" And I tell them, "I don't care what it is—just give me three things."

It doesn't have to be profound; it can be as simple as a paperclip holding their papers together, the stairs in their home helping them get up and down, or even the fact that their morning coffee didn't spill on the way to work. One client told me she was grateful for the extra five minutes she got to snooze her alarm, while another said he was thankful for the perfectly ripe banana he had for breakfast. Someone else mentioned being grateful for the sound of rain, which made them feel cozy, even on a tough day. The point is, gratitude doesn't have to be grand—it just has to be acknowledged.

On those really challenging days when life feels like it's piling up, digging deep for gratitude can make all the difference. It's about finding those little sparks of positivity, even when they seem buried. So when I ask for three things, don't overthink it—just take a moment, breathe, and find those small blessings that might otherwise go unnoticed. Trust me, it's a game-changer.

And while keeping a gratitude journal isn't mandatory, I highly recommend it.

Writing down what you're grateful for each day can really help solidify this practice and keep your mindset in a positive place, even on the toughest days. Give it a try—you might be surprised at how powerful this simple habit can be.

Here are some strategies to enhance your sense of gratitude:

- Notice the Little Things: Maybe it's the smell of your morning coffee, a kind word from a colleague, or even a moment of peace.

- Pause and Reflect: Take a moment during your day to acknowledge and savor the goodness around you.

- Use a Gratitude App or Journal: These tools can prompt you to regularly reflect on the blessings in your life.

- Express It Out Loud: Let people know when you appreciate something they've done. It not only makes their day, but it also strengthens your own sense of gratitude.

Embracing gratitude not only enriches your personal experience but also helps you build a deeper sense of contentment and connection with the world around you. So grab that journal, and start celebrating the small wins—every single one of them!

4. *Get Ready, Get Set, Almost There...Just Gotta Download The REBOOT Guide: Scan QR Code To Download The REBOOT Guide*

Alright, REBOOTERS, let's talk about the one tool you absolutely "must" keep by your side as you embark on this journey—the REBOOT Guide. Think of it as your trusty sidekick, your go-to resource, and the ultimate cheat sheet for everything you'll need during the RESET. This isn't just a bunch of pages stapled together; it's packed with everything from a "RESET At A Glance" chart to keep you on track, to anti-inflammatory, low-sugar recipes that are as tasty as they are healthy. Here's a little secret—it's also included in the back of the book, but it might be easier to keep a separate copy handy as a reference in the kitchen or wherever you need it most.

Feeling snacky? No problem! The REBOOT Guide has you covered with smart snacking ideas, high-protein options, and grab-n-go bites that'll satisfy your cravings without sabotaging your progress. Got a sweet tooth? Don't worry—I've included some sweet treats that won't derail your journey.

But wait, there's more! The Guide also includes a pantry list to help you stock up on essentials, and even a list of anti-inflammatory baking staples for all you bakers out there.

So, keep your REBOOT Guide close—it's like having a nutritionist, a chef, and a motivational coach all rolled into one. Now, let's dive in and make this RESET as smooth and successful as possible!

5. **Get Ready, Get Set, Almost There....Is My Pantry REBOOT Ready?...Stocking Your Pantry**

Before you dive into the exciting changes ahead, it's time to make sure your kitchen is fully prepped for success. Trust me, you don't want to be caught in a snack emergency without the right foods on hand! So, grab your REBOOT Guide and take a good, long look at the pantry list. This isn't just a casual suggestion—it's a crucial step in getting you ready to crush this journey.

As the wise Benjamin Franklin once said, "By failing to prepare, you are preparing to fail." Let's make sure that's not you. Being ready means having your pantry stocked with all the delicious, anti-inflammatory foods you'll be including in your diet. No more standing in front of the fridge, wondering what on earth you can eat.

But don't worry—stocking up doesn't have to break the bank. There are plenty of resources for affordable, healthy, and organic foods that can be delivered right to your front door, like Misfit Market and Thrive Market. Plus, you can find great deals at Target, Amazon, Costco, and Aldi. They all offer some fantastic finds that will keep your pantry filled without emptying your wallet.

You've already done the hard work—your mojo is in check, your measurements and photos are done, you've started your gratitude journal, and you've downloaded your REBOOT Guide. Now, it's time for the fun part: shopping! Head out (or online) and fill your cart with all the amazing foods that are going to fuel your transformation. After all, if you're going to REBOOT your life, you might as well do it with a fully stocked pantry and a confident smile. Let's get shopping and set yourself up for success!

6. Get Ready, Get Set, You're Ready To Go!

Alright, you're all set! You've got your REBOOT Guide in hand, your pantry stocked with all the good stuff, and a mindset ready for success. Now it's time to dive into this RESET with confidence. Remember, this journey is about progress, not perfection—so take it one day at a time, and don't sweat the small stuff.

But hey, if you have a bad day, don't throw in the towel. Just keep going! My motto is "Progress Over Perfection"— because this is a journey, not a sprint. I have total faith in you, and I know you can do this! You're stronger than you think, and the commitment you've made to yourself is already half the battle won. So, take a deep breath, trust the process, and let's get this REBOOT started. You've got this!

Chapter 4: Cracking The Food Code
The RESET

Welcome to "Cracking The Food Code," where we unlock the secrets to optimal health by kicking out the foods that wreak havoc on your gut and body. Now that you've got a grip on the basics from the REBOOT, it's time to jump into the RESET—a 21-day journey to heal your body by eliminating inflammatory foods. Trust me, those pesky symptoms like rashes, joint pain, headaches, fatigue, bloating, and sleep issues, sound familiar? They often trace back to gut inflammation and a microbial imbalance (basically, when the bad guys outnumber the good guys in your gut).

Your gut is home to about 100 trillion bacteria, outnumbering your body's cells by a landslide. When the bad bacteria take over, it can lead to chronic and autoimmune diseases. The good news? You can give your gut a major upgrade just by changing what you eat. The RESET is all about gradually eliminating different foods every three days, giving your body a chance to heal and your gut a chance to thrive. And here's the kicker—once you remove a food, it's out for the rest of the RESET. No cheating!

Ready to get started? If you haven't already, download your REBOOT Guide by scanning the QR code in the "Chapter 3, Getting Started Section", or refer to the back of the book. It's packed with a "RESET at a Glance" timeline, meal ideas, a handy anti-inflammatory pantry list, and REBOOT-approved recipes—basically, everything you need to crush this 21-day journey and come out feeling healthier and more balanced than ever!

At the end of each RESET section you will find a set of "guidelines". These guidelines are your roadmap to healthier habits, laying the foundation for better overall health. By following these steps, you're taking a crucial step toward reducing inflammation, supporting heart health, and fueling your body with the right kind of foods it needs to thrive. Remember, these aren't just suggestions; they are actionable steps designed to help you achieve your best health. Stick to them, revisit them, and let them guide your choices in the kitchen every day. Your body will thank you for it!

Days 1-21: Meat & Alcohol RESET

Why RESET Meat?

Let's face it—meat, especially the red and processed kind, isn't doing your body any favors. Research shows that goodies like bacon, hot dogs, jerky, pepperoni, salami, and sausages are major players in the inflammation game. And if that wasn't bad enough, higher intakes of these meats are linked to some pretty scary stuff like cancer, heart disease, and stroke—all of which have inflammation written all over them. Processed meats are also loaded with nitrates, which have been linked to diabetes, faster aging, and—you guessed it—cancer. Plus, eating conventionally raised meat could be messing with your hormone levels, especially estrogen. Whether it's the hormones in the meat, the gut bacteria of those who eat it, or a combo of both, too much meat can throw your hormones out of whack by boosting estrogen production.

Why should you care? Well, estrogen dominance can lead to conditions like diabetes, metabolic syndrome, PCOS, and certain types of cancer. One way to keep your estrogen in check is by upping your fiber intake. Fiber not only helps reduce estrogen levels but also protects against some cancers. It's like your body's little cleanup crew, sweeping out excess estrogen and keeping your gut and hormones in balance. But that's not all—conventional and processed meats can expose you to toxins. The Environmental Working Group (EWG) found that a hefty percentage of beef, pork, and turkey might contain superbugs thanks to the overuse of antibiotics in farming. These superbugs are bacteria and other nasties that resist most antibiotics, making them a real problem. Add in the cocktail of steroid hormones, persistent organic pollutants (POPs), and GMO grain feed, and you've got a recipe for inflammation, hormone disruption, and a leaky gut.

Leaky gut sounds gross, right? That's because it is. It happens when your gut lining gets too thin, letting harmful toxins slip into your bloodstream. This can lead to inflammation and all sorts of health issues. Plus, toxins stored in the fat of conventionally raised animals can make their way to your liver and bloodstream, potentially causing obesity, insulin resistance, and cancer.

Now, ***don't panic***—we're not saying you can never eat meat again! But for now, we're going to hit the pause button on red meat and all those cured, fermented, processed, and smoked varieties. Later, when we're ready to refuel our diets, we'll explore healthier meat options that won't leave you missing a thing.

What Can You Eat?

Substitute other protein sources such as pasture-raised chicken, turkey, duck, and eggs; lentils; organic tofu (not soy isolate); wild-caught cold-water fish; shellfish and crustaceans; pea-based protein powder; healthy fats; nut butters; and seeds.

Meat Reset Guidelines:

- REMOVE all red meat and cured, fermented, and smoked meats.
    - Red meat includes beef, pork, lamb, veal, mutton, goat, and venison.

- REMOVE all processed meat.
    - Sausages, hot dogs, salami
    - Ham, cured bacon
    - Salted and cured meat, corned beef
    - Smoked meat
    - Dried meat, beef jerky
    - Canned meat

- INCLUDE:4-6 ounces of protein per meal:
    - Pasture-raised chicken, turkey, and duck
    - Pasture-raised eggs
    - Lentils
    - Organic tofu (not soy isolate)
    - Wild-caught cold-water fish
    - Shellfish and crustaceans
    - Pea-based protein powder
    - Healthy fats
    - Nut butters and seeds

- Gradually increase your vegetable intake to at least 3 to 4 cups per day:

- Include both raw and cooked vegetables.
- A serving is a cup of raw or half a cup of cooked vegetables.
- Buy local, fresh, and organic when you can to cut back on toxins.
- Refer to the EWG list of healthy/clean vegetables:

Refer to https://www.ewg.org/foodnews/ for more information!

- Gradually increase your fiber intake by 5 grams per day until you reach the American Heart Association's recommended range of 25g-30g per day:
  - Track your total fiber intake to ensure you are getting at least 25g-30g per day; supplement if needed with a combination of soluble and insoluble fiber.

- Stay hydrated
  - Ensure you are drinking plenty of water throughout the day to support your overall health and the RESET process.

Why Do We RESET Alcohol? —WAIT…PLEASE DON'T STOP HERE!

I know the mere thought of giving up alcohol for a few weeks might have you reconsidering this whole thing. Trust me, I get it! I love a good martini or a nice glass of wine just as much as the next person. But here's the deal—between my autoimmune disease and menopause, my tolerance for alcohol has taken a nosedive. Yep, menopause can do that! Who knew? Whether you're a man or a woman, research shows plenty of good reasons to cut back on the booze, and there are some real benefits to doing so. So, let me ask you this: Do you want to burn fat, improve your sleep, and clear the cobwebs out of your brain, or are you content with that "nightcap" we've all grown so fond of to "wind down" after a long day? I'm not saying you can never have alcohol again (because I know some of you are eyeing the exit right now). But I am asking you to give your metabolism a much-needed RESET by taking a break for the next 21 days. After all, it's just three weeks—you've got this!

Facts About Alcohol Consumption

Let's be real—if alcohol had a resume, it would probably include "Life of the Party" at the top. But before you invite it to all your events, let's talk about some of the not-so-great things that come with it. You know, the side effects that make you wish you'd left the party early!

Drinking too much alcohol, whether occasionally or regularly, can have serious health consequences. Alcohol is a neurotoxin, meaning it can harm your brain, potentially leading to memory problems, strokes, multiple sclerosis, and even Alzheimer's disease. It also messes with how your brain communicates, which can affect your mood and behavior. Your heart isn't safe either—excessive drinking can lead to heart problems like cardiomyopathy (a disease of the heart muscle), irregular heartbeat, stroke, and high blood pressure. The liver also takes a hit, with risks of fatty liver, alcoholic hepatitis, fibrosis, and cirrhosis.

Alcohol doesn't stop there. It can damage your pancreas, leading to pancreatitis and digestion issues. It weakens your immune system, making you more vulnerable to infections for up to 24 hours after drinking. The National Cancer Institute has linked alcohol to higher risks of several cancers, including those of the head, neck, esophagus, liver, breast, and colon.

Alcohol also raises cortisol levels, which can increase your appetite and cause cravings for unhealthy foods, leading to weight gain. Plus, it disrupts gut health, causing an imbalance in gut bacteria (dysbiosis) that can lead to inflammation and conditions like Leaky Gut Syndrome. In short, drinking too much alcohol can lead to a range of health problems, making moderation key to staying healthy.

Alcohol Guidelines

Alright, let's talk about alcohol guidelines—because, let's be honest, no one wants to be that person Googling, "How much wine is "too" much wine?"

According to the CDC, moderate drinking means one drink per day for women and two for men. Now, before you start negotiating with yourself ("Does that mean I can save up all my drinks for Saturday?"), let's be clear: you can't hoard your weekly drink allowance and unleash it all in one night. That's not how moderation works! Sure, a little wine now and then might have some perks—hello, antioxidants!—but trying to squeeze a week's worth of "moderation" into one wild night? That's where the trouble starts. So, let's keep it classy, folks. Enjoy that glass of wine, but maybe leave the bottle for another day. Your liver—and your future self—will thank you!

Days 4-21: The Sugar RESET

Cutting sugar from your diet is like trying to break up with that charming but totally unreliable ex—you know it's the right thing to do, but somehow they keep showing up everywhere! You start the day with the best intentions, thinking, "Today is the day! No sugar for me!" But then lunchtime rolls around, and there's that innocent-looking muffin, batting its sugary eyelashes at you. And let's not even talk about the sneaky sugar hiding in your favorite salad dressing. Before you know it, you're making excuses like, "It's just a little treat," or "I'll start fresh tomorrow."

But here's the thing: just like with that ex, the longer you keep sugar around, the harder it is to imagine life without it. Breaking up is tough, but with a little willpower—and maybe a few savory snacks on standby—you can finally give sugar the boot. And who knows? You might just find that life without the sugar rollercoaster feels pretty damn good!

Why RESET Sugar?

Removing sugar from your diet is tough, but once you do it, you'll wonder why you didn't make the change sooner! *A Sugar RESET* is crucial for reducing inflammation and kickstarting weight loss. Yes, it might feel like you're saying goodbye to your best friend, but trust me, there are plenty of amazing foods and snacks out there that are low in sugar yet still bursting with flavor. You won't even miss the sugary stuff! Check out the REBOOT Guide for some mouthwatering ideas.

Now, let's get into the details: What's the difference between natural sugar, added sugar, and fructose? And how do they affect our hormones, metabolism, and inflammation? Spoiler alert: understanding these differences is key to mastering your Sugar RESET and keeping your health on track!

Natural Sugar, aka "The Boring Sugar"

Naturally occurring sugars are found in foods such as milk and fruit and have not been linked to inflammation. In fact, many foods containing natural sugars, such as fruits and vegetables, may be anti-inflammatory and contain other nutrients such as protein and fiber.

Added Sugar: The Sneaky Saboteur

Let's talk about added sugar—the sneaky stuff that finds its way into your food when you're not looking. Added sugars are those extra sweeteners mixed into food during preparation, long before it hits your plate. You will spot them in the usual suspects like sugary drinks, desserts, candy, and even in that sweetened coffee you adore. But here's the kicker: added sugar is hiding in more places than you'd expect! In fact, three out of four products on grocery store shelves have added sugar, making it a real challenge to dodge them.

To make matters trickier, added sugar can go by 61 different names on food labels. Yep, 61! When it comes to understanding sugar's many hidden forms in our food, it's crucial to stay informed. Laura Schmidt, PhD, MSW, MPH, a professor of health policy at the University of California, San Francisco, and her team at SugarScience.org, have made it their mission to educate the public about these sugar aliases. This initiative is particularly important, as the FDA's updated food labeling is helping, but there are still many sugar disguises out there. For more information on hidden sugars and their impact on health, visit [SugarScience.org](https:// sugarscience.ucsf.edu/) or check out the FDA's guidelines on food labeling. These resources can help you make more informed choices and better understand the sugars in your diet.

Here's a comprehensive list of the 61 names for sugar, so you can spot
"hidden sugars" in your food:

Agave nectar, Barbados sugar, Barley malt, Barley malt syrup, Beet sugar, Brown sugar, Buttered syrup, Cane juice, Cane juice crystals, Cane sugar, Caramel, Carob syrup, Castor sugar, Coconut palm sugar, Coconut sugar, Confectioner's sugar, Corn sweetener, Corn syrup, Corn syrup solids, Date sugar, Dehydrated cane juice, Demerara sugar, Dextrin, Dextrose, Evaporated cane juice, Free-flowing brown sugars, Fructose, Fruit juice, Fruit juice concentrate, Glucose, Glucose solids, Golden sugar, Golden syrup, Grape sugar, HFCS (high-fructose corn syrup), Honey, Icing sugar, Invert sugar, Malt syrup, Maltodextrin, Maltol, Maltose, Mannose, Maple syrup, Molasses, Muscovado, Palm sugar, Panocha, Powdered sugar, Raw sugar, Refiner's syrup, Rice syrup, Saccharose, Sorghum syrup, Sucrose, Sugar (granulated), Sweet sorghum, Syrup, Treacle, Turbinado sugar, Yellow sugar.

When you eat foods with added sugars, the sugar enters your bloodstream, and your body releases insulin to help convert that sugar into energy. But if there's too much sugar, the extra gets stored in your fat cells, causing them to get larger. Over time, this can lead to weight gain and insulin resistance—the point when your body stops responding to insulin as it should. Insulin resistance is linked to conditions like type 2 diabetes and metabolic syndrome, and it's a major player in chronic inflammation.

And so begins the vicious cycle; more sugar means more insulin, which means more fat storage, leading to inflammation, and around we go.

Feeling overwhelmed yet? Don't worry—the good news is that cutting out added sugar can help break this cycle. Your cravings will ease up, your insulin levels will stabilize, and you might even find yourself not missing sugar at all. It might sound as believable as a unicorn doing your laundry, but trust me, it happens. Many of my clients start out skeptical, and then a few weeks later, they're amazed at how little they crave sugar. It's like their taste buds took a vacation and came back refreshed! It might feel like a daunting task, but remember, slow and steady wins the race. Soon enough, you'll be breezing past the cookie aisle like a pro!

Fructose: The Sweet but Sneaky Sugar

Fructose is a natural sugar found in fruits, fruit juices, and honey—so far, so good, right? But here's where it gets tricky: fructose also makes up about half of table sugar (sucrose). While the fructose in whole fruits is totally fine (go ahead, eat that apple!), the fructose in table sugar and sweeteners like high fructose corn syrup is a different story.

Fructose is about 73% sweeter than table sugar, which is why it's found in sweeteners like agave and, you guessed it, high fructose corn syrup. Now, while glucose (the other half of table sugar) is used by your body for energy right away, fructose has to take a detour through the liver, where it's converted into glucose. Sounds simple enough, but here's the catch: if you're consuming too much fructose, your liver can't keep up. Instead of being turned into glucose, the excess gets converted into fat, which then makes its way into your bloodstream as triglycerides or gets stashed in your liver and belly.

But wait, *there's more!* Some folks can't absorb all the fructose they eat (hello, fructose malabsorption), leading to gas and digestive discomfort—not exactly a fun time. And just like too much glucose can mess with your insulin, too much fructose can mess with leptin, the hormone that tells your brain you're full. When your brain doesn't get the memo to stop eating, you keep munching away, leading to leptin resistance, where your brain is basically ignoring the "I'm full" signal. This can contribute to that pesky low-grade inflammation we're all trying to avoid. *So yes, it's exhausting and unfair*—kind of like trying to avoid spoilers for your favorite TV show. But hang in there, **you're doing great!**

Sugar and Chronic Disease: The Not-So-Sweet Truth

We all love a bit of sweetness in our lives, but when it comes to sugar, too much of a good thing can lead to some serious health issues. Research has shown that a high intake of added sugars and refined carbs is linked to a buffet of chronic diseases—heart disease, cancer, diabetes, obesity, and more.

Let's break it down: added sugar is a major culprit in the obesity epidemic, which is now recognized as a low-grade inflammatory disease. This inflammation also ramps up the risk of type 2 diabetes, high blood pressure, and heart disease. The connection? Sugar fuels low-grade inflammation, which is the sneaky link between sugar and chronic diseases. Then there's fructose, the sugar found in many sweetened foods and drinks. When you consume too much fructose, it messes with your blood lipids, causes fat to accumulate in your liver, and can lead to insulin resistance. This nasty trio can result in obesity and type 2 diabetes.

So, How Much Sugar Are We Really Eating?

Brace yourself... according to the CDC, between 2017 and 2018, the average American adult was consuming 17-18 teaspoons of added sugar each day. That's a lot of sugar! No wonder the U.S. is a world leader in sugar consumption and ranks third globally in sugary drink sales. Unfortunately, this also puts the U.S. at the top of the list for obesity rates, including childhood obesity—a statistic that's *anything but sweet*. In 2021, more than 38 million Americans had diabetes, with 90-95% of these cases being type 2 diabetes. And the numbers are only going up.

According to the latest stats,
"An American is diagnosed with diabetes every 17 seconds."

But here's the good news: type 2 diabetes is largely preventable and can be managed with a healthy diet and regular exercise. Reducing your sugar intake is a key step in lowering inflammation, preventing weight gain, and reducing your risk of developing type 2 diabetes.

The American Heart Association (AHA) recommends that men keep their added sugar intake to no more than 9 teaspoons (38 grams) per day, and women should aim for no more than 6 teaspoons (25 grams) per day. So, next time you reach for that sugary treat, just remember—a little less sugar can go a long way in keeping your health on track!

Sugar Reset Guidelines:

- Aim for the AHA recommendation of no more than 6 teaspoons (25 grams) of added sugar per day for women, and 9 teaspoons (38 grams) for men.
- Remove all sugar substitutes and artificial sweeteners. *Stevia or Monk Fruit* are the only acceptable sugar alternatives.
- REMOVE ALL HIGH FRUCTOSE CORN SYRUP.

- Remove honey, agave nectar, and table sugar (see complete list above)
- Limit fruit juice to 4 oz. per day.
- Eat 3 to 4+ cups of vegetables per day; some cooked and some raw (dark green leafy vegetables are best).
- Try to get 25 to 30 grams of fiber per day.
- Include low-glycemic fruits such as: berries, cherries, plums, apples, pears, oranges, grapefruit
- Choose low-glycemic grains such as: quinoa, buckwheat, wild rice, steel-cut oats, and millet.
- Include 4 to 6 oz. of clean protein at each meal: pasture-raised chicken, pasture-raised eggs, lentils, organic tofu (not soy isolate), wild-caught cold-water fish, shellfish and crustaceans, pea-based protein powder, healthy fats, nut butters, and seeds.

Days 7-21: Refined Fats and Oils RESET

Let's Talk About the "F" Word...

Got your attention, didn't I? For years, Americans were led to believe that all fats were the enemy, thanks to outdated dietary guidelines that pushed low-fat diets as the solution to heart disease and weight management. This fat phobia led many to avoid it entirely, opting instead for low-fat, processed products that were often packed with sugar and refined carbs. But here's the thing: not all fats are created equal, and it's time to set the record straight. In fact, "healthy fats" are like the superheroes of your diet. Found in foods like avocados, nuts, seeds, olive oil, and fatty fish, these beneficial fats are crucial for keeping your brain sharp, your heart healthy, and your inflammation in check.

So, instead of running from fat like it's the villain in a horror movie, it's important to distinguish between the unhealthy fats and those that can actually give your health a boost. Incorporating healthy fats into your diet can lead to better energy levels, improved nutrient absorption, and a lower risk of chronic diseases.

The takeaway? Not all fats are the same. Some are your body's best friend, helping to fuel your energy and fight inflammation, while others—not so much. The key is knowing which fats are the good guys, so you can keep your body running like a well-oiled machine (pun intended!).

Trans Fats vs. Saturated Fats: The Battle of the Bad Guys

Let's clear up the confusion about these two types of fats—because while they sound similar, they're like the evil twins of the fat world, each with its own set of problems.

Trans Fats are the real troublemakers. They're created through hydrogenation, a process that turns healthy oils into solids to keep them from spoiling. Sounds handy, right? Well, not so much. Studies have shown that eating trans fats can lead to heart disease, inflammation, and mess up your cholesterol by raising the bad (LDL) and lowering the good (HDL). Trans fats are so bad that many of them have been banned in the U.S., but you might still find them lurking in things like vegetable shortening, margarine, and some vegetable oils. If you see "partially hydrogenated oils" on the label, it's best to put that product back on the shelf and walk away.

Saturated Fats are a bit more complicated. You'll find them in animal-based foods like beef, pork, poultry, full-fat dairy products, and tropical oils like coconut and palm oil.

Saturated fats have been in the hot seat since the 1950s, with debates raging over whether they cause heart disease. While it's true that they can raise your cholesterol, recent research has shown that they may not be as evil as once thought—at least for most healthy adults. However, *not all saturated fats are created equal*. The kind found in whole foods like milk, cheese, and yogurt might not be as harmful as those found in processed meats and sugary treats. But don't go buttering your bread with reckless abandon just yet. Both the American Heart Association and the World Health Organization still recommend limiting your intake of saturated fats. If you're watching your LDL cholesterol, aim to keep your saturated fat intake to 5-6% of your total calories. So, while a little fat can be part of a healthy diet, moderation is key!

OMEGA-3 and OMEGA-6 FATTY ACIDS—
Omega-3 vs. Omega-6: The Fatty Acid Showdown

Let's talk about Omega-3 and Omega-6 fatty acids—the two types of polyunsaturated fats that your body absolutely needs but can't make on its own. Yep, you've got to get these bad boys from your diet, which is why they're called "essential" fatty acids. Unlike other fats, these guys are more than just energy sources—they're biologically active and play key roles in your body's functions.

Omega-3s are the superstars of the fat world, with benefits that read like a health nut's dream list. You can find them in fatty fish like salmon, mackerel, herring, and sardines, as well as in plant sources like flaxseeds, chia seeds, and walnuts. These fats are linked to all sorts of good stuff: boosting brain and heart health, reducing inflammation, preventing dangerous blood clots, lowering triglycerides, balancing blood sugar, helping manage autoimmune diseases, and protecting against a slew of chronic illnesses. Basically, they're the fat equivalent of a superhero cape.

Omega-6s have their perks too, but they're a bit more controversial. You'll find them in oils like safflower, sunflower, corn, and soybean, as well as in sunflower seeds, walnuts, and pumpkin seeds. The problem is that the Standard American Diet (*SAD—aptly named, right?*) is loaded with Omega-6s, thanks to the processed foods packed with seed and vegetable oils. Ideally, your Omega-6 to Omega-3 ratio should be around 1:1, or maybe 4:1 at worst. But with the SAD, that ratio can skyrocket to about 16:1! That's like inviting way too many guests to a party—things get out of hand fast. For years, Omega-6s were the bad guys of the fat world, but not all of them are evil. They can help lower bad cholesterol (LDL), boost good cholesterol (HDL), and regulate blood sugar. The goal isn't to banish Omega-6s from your diet but to balance them out with more Omega-3s. Get those two in harmony, and your body will thank you!

So, What's the Recommendation?

The American Heart Association and the Institute of Medicine suggest that 5-10% of your daily calories should come from Omega-6 fats. *But here's the catch:* most Americans are getting way more Omega-6s than Omega-3s—like ten times more. And that imbalance isn't doing your heart any favors. The solution? Don't slash those healthy Omega-6 fats from your diet; instead, pump up your intake of Omega-3s to even the score.

Wondering where to find those Omega-3s? Look no further than fatty fish like anchovies, salmon, mackerel, sardines, and herring, which are all excellent sources. If you're feeling adventurous, cod liver oil is another option, and for those moments when you're feeling fancy, oysters and caviar also pack a punch. For a plant-based boost, flaxseed and chia seeds make great smoothie additions, while walnuts are perfect for snacking. Even soybeans can help you get your Omega-3 fix if you're a tofu lover. With so many tasty options, it's easy to incorporate Omega-3s into your diet. But if these foods don't quite do it for you, consider chatting with a Registered Dietitian or your healthcare provider about adding an Omega-3 supplement to your routine—your heart will thank you!

Butter vs. Better Fats: What's the Scoop?

Butter has long been the subject of debate in the nutrition world. On one hand, it's a great source of vitamin A and vitamin E, both of which help protect your cells from damage. Butter also contains conjugated linoleic acid (CLA), known for its potential to aid in fat loss, improve immune function, and even offer anti-cancer properties. And let's not forget butyrate—a short-chain fatty acid in butter that supports gut health and reduces inflammation, making it a powerful ally for those managing IBS or Crohn's Disease.

Now, if you're reaching for butter, grass-fed is your best bet. Compared to its conventional counterpart, grass-fed butter packs more vitamin K2 and Omega-3 fatty acids. In moderation, it can certainly be part of a healthy diet, but if you're monitoring your LDL (bad) cholesterol, the American Heart Association suggests switching to heart-healthy plant fats like avocado or olive oil.

Speaking of olive oil, this should be the number one cooking oil in your kitchen! Research consistently shows that olive oil boasts anti-inflammatory benefits, thanks to its rich antioxidant content. It's been proven to improve circulation, boost the immune system, promote gut health, and reduce inflammation. To get the most bang for your buck, opt for the best quality olive oil your budget allows—extra-virgin, cold-pressed, and organic when possible.

Avocado oil is another excellent option, particularly for high-heat cooking. It's rich in monounsaturated fats and offers anti-inflammatory and heart health benefits. And don't forget about coconut oil and ghee—both have their own set of perks. Coconut oil, for instance, has potential anti-inflammatory and antibacterial properties, while ghee is packed with vitamins A and D and contains more monounsaturated fats.

In summary, while butter—especially grass-fed—has its place, diversifying your fats with high-quality olive oil, avocado oil, and even coconut oil or ghee is a smart move for your overall health. Your body will thank you for it!

Fats <u>NOT</u> to Use

Let's keep it simple: when it comes to fats, some are great for you, while others are better left on the shelf. The problem with certain oils—like corn, soybean, canola (rapeseed), cottonseed, rice bran, safflower, and sunflower—is that they're often processed at high temperatures and treated with chemicals. This processing damages the fats, leading to something called "oxidative stress" in your body, which can cause inflammation—exactly what you don't want. These oils are common in processed foods and restaurant dishes, but they're not doing your body any favors. Think of them as the

76

bad guys in your diet—sneaky, harmful, and best avoided. Instead, stick to healthier fats, and your body will thank you!

Include Foods Rich In "Healthy Fats"

- **Avocados**
  - Rich in monounsaturated fats
  - Contains fiber, potassium, and vitamins C, E, and K

- **Olive Oil, Extra Virgin, Cold-Pressed** (organic)
  - High in monounsaturated fats, particularly oleic acid
  - Contains antioxidants and anti-inflammatory properties

- **Nuts**
  - Almonds: High in monounsaturated fats, fiber, vitamin E, and magnesium
  - Walnuts: Rich in omega-3 fatty acids, antioxidants, and polyunsaturated fats
  - Pistachios: Contains monounsaturated fats, fiber, and protein
  - Macadamia Nuts: Very high in monounsaturated fats, with a good amount of fiber and minerals

- **Seeds**
  - Chia Seeds: Rich in omega-3 fatty acids, fiber, and protein
  - Flaxseeds: High in omega-3 fatty acids, lignans, and fiber
  - Hemp Seeds: Contains a balanced ratio of omega-3 and omega-6 fatty acids, along with protein
  - Pumpkin Seeds: High in monounsaturated fats, magnesium, and antioxidants

- **Fatty Fish**
  - Salmon Rich in omega-3 fatty acids (EPA and DHA), protein, and B vitamins
  - Mackerel: High in omega-3 fatty acids, vitamin D, and selenium
  - Sardines: Contains omega-3 fatty acids, calcium, and vitamin D
  - Trout: High in omega-3 fatty acids and vitamin D

- **Dark Chocolate**
  - Contains monounsaturated fats, flavonoids, and antioxidants
  - Choose dark chocolate with 70% cocoa or higher for the most benefits

- **Coconut Oil**
  - High in medium-chain triglycerides (MCTs), which are easily digestible and can be used for energy
  - Contains lauric acid, which has antimicrobial properties

- **Full-Fat Dairy**
  - Greek Yogurt: High in protein, calcium, and probiotics, with healthy fats in full-fat versions
  - Cheese: Contains conjugated linoleic acid (CLA), calcium, and protein
  - Butter: Particularly from grass-fed cows, high in butyrate and omega-3 fatty acids

- **Eggs**
  - Especially from pastured or omega-3 enriched chickens
  - Contains healthy fats, protein, vitamins, and minerals

- **Olives**
  - High in monounsaturated fats, especially oleic acid
  - Contains antioxidants, including vitamin E

- **Nut Butters**
  - Almond Butter: Rich in monounsaturated fats, vitamin E, and magnesium
  - Peanut Butter: Contains monounsaturated fats and protein (choose natural, with no added sugars or oils)
  - Cashew Butter: High in monounsaturated fats, copper, and magnesium

- **Ghee (Clarified Butter)**
  - High in saturated fats, particularly butyrate
  - Contains fat-soluble vitamins A, D, E, and K

- **Organic Tofu and Tempeh**
  - Made from soybeans, which contain polyunsaturated fats, particularly omega-3 fatty acids
  - Also a good source of protein and fiber

These foods are excellent sources of healthy fats that can be incorporated into a balanced diet to support overall health and well-being.

Refined Oils & Fat Guidelines:

- STOP using refined oils such as corn, soybean, rapeseed/canola, cottonseed, rice bran, safflower, and sunflower oils.
- AVOID products made with trans fats (partially hydrogenated oils).
- CHOOSE olive and avocado oils for cooking.
- INCLUDE foods rich in healthy fats.
- Aim for at least two servings per week of foods that are high in Omega-3 fatty acids.
- LIMIT saturated fats to less than 10 percent of total caloric intake.
- Switch to grass-fed butter when consuming butter.

Days 10-21: Gluten, Grains & Inflammation—The GRAIN-FREE RESET

Carbs often get a bad rap, kind of like the "F" word we discussed earlier. While foods high in "complex" carbohydrates can be nutritious and an important part of a balanced diet, it's the "simple carbs"—especially those made from refined grains —that can stir up trouble. These sneaky little devils are like the party crashers of your diet, showing up uninvited, causing chaos, and leaving a mess behind. They can ramp up inflammation, encourage the growth of bad gut bacteria, and increase your risk of inflammatory diseases. Refined grains are basically the fast food of the grain world. They've had their bran and germ removed, leaving only the endosperm behind— think of it as taking a juicy, nutrient-packed apple and stripping it down to just the sugary core. This process removes all the good stuff—dietary fiber, iron, and B vitamins—leaving you with a product that raises your blood sugar faster than you can say, "insulin spike!" And when your blood sugar shoots up, so does your insulin, leading to fat storage and all the joys that come with it. It's like riding a blood sugar rollercoaster, except without the fun part.

Then there's gluten, the protein found in wheat. For some, it's not just a bread-and-butter issue—it's more like a bread-and-butter betrayal. Gluten can be a real inflammation trigger, turning your favorite foods into a not-so-fun surprise for your gut.

Refined carbohydrates are lurking in all your favorite indulgences—candy, bread, pasta, pastries, cereals, cookies, cakes, sugary soft drinks, and pretty much any processed food with added sugar or flour. They're hard to avoid, but cutting them out during your Grain-Free Reset can help reduce inflammation and improve your overall health. And who knows? You might just find that life without those refined grains is a lot tastier than you thought!

Before we talk about how to cut them out, let's take a closer look at what a typical day on the Standard American Diet, loaded with refined grains, often looks like. Spoiler alert: it's a rollercoaster of quick fixes and energy crashes! From breakfast to late-night snacks, let's dive into a day where convenience and carbs reign supreme.

A Day in the Life on the Standard American Diet: **The Refined Grains Edition**

Morning:
The alarm blares at 6:30 AM, and there's no time to waste. Breakfast? That's whatever's quickest—a couple of slices of white toast smothered in butter or a bowl of sugary cereal will do the trick. Paired with a large coffee that's more cream and sugar than actual coffee, this breakfast sets the day in motion. The refined grains and sugar offer a quick burst of energy, but it's the kind of energy that burns out faster than you can say "breakfast."

Mid-Morning:
By 10:00 AM, the stomach is already growling again, and the office break room beckons. A muffin or a granola bar (which is really just a candy bar in disguise) seems like the perfect pick-me-up. Unfortunately, these snacks are packed with refined grains and sugars, leading to another short-lived energy boost followed by the inevitable mid-morning slump.

Lunch:

Lunchtime arrives, and it's all about convenience. A sandwich made with white bread, a side of chips, and maybe a soda to wash it down—classic lunch fare. It's filling, sure, but high in refined grains, unhealthy fats, and sugars. The meal leaves a sense of fullness that quickly turns into sluggishness, making the rest of the afternoon feel like a chore.

Afternoon:

Around 3:00 PM, energy levels plummet again, and another snack is needed to make it through the day. A handful of crackers or a slice of leftover pizza—both loaded with refined grains—seem like easy choices. The quick carbs provide an instant pick-me-up, but it's short-lived, leading to yet another energy crash.

Dinner:

As dinner rolls around, the trend of quick fixes continues. A plate of pasta made with white noodles, some garlic bread on the side, and a pre-made sauce loaded with added sugars is the meal of choice. It's another satisfying but nutritionally lacking meal, dominated by refined grains that continue the cycle of energy spikes and crashes.

Evening:

The day winds down, and it's time for a little late-night snacking. A bowl of popcorn or another slice of white bread toast seems like the perfect thing to nibble on while unwinding in front of the TV. These snacks, filled with refined carbs, offer comfort but little in the way of nutritional value.

End of Day:

As the day comes to a close, the body feels heavy, tired, and strangely unsatisfied despite the constant intake of food. It's been a day filled with meals and snacks high in refined grains, sugars, and unhealthy fats—foods that provide quick energy but leave the body craving more, setting the stage for a repeat performance tomorrow.

Sound familiar?

When your diet is loaded with refined grains, it's like fueling your body with cheap gas—you might get by for a while, but eventually, things start to break down. Refined grains, stripped of their fiber and nutrients, cause rapid spikes and crashes in blood sugar, leaving you constantly hungry and more likely to overeat. This cycle contributes to poor health and is a major driver of the obesity epidemic in the U.S. Let's explore how this diet, with its lack of real nutrients and reliance on quick fixes, is wreaking havoc on our health...and our waist!

The Standard American Diet (SAD) and OBESITY: A Recipe for Disaster

The Standard American Diet, often called "SAD," is an acronym that couldn't be more fitting if it tried. In a world where convenience is king, we've traded in nutrition for fast food drive-thrus, sugary drinks, and snacks that are more about instant gratification than actual nourishment. Sure, they fill you up in the short term, but over time, they leave your body feeling like it's running on fumes.

As a society, we've mastered the art of supersizing everything—portions, fries, you name it. Our meals are often more about satisfying our immediate cravings than thinking about what's good for us in the long run. And let's be real, who hasn't been tempted by the lure of something quick and greasy when the day's been long and the couch is calling? But those choices add up, and *not* in a good way.

What's the result? A slow but steady march toward an obesity epidemic that's spreading across the U.S. like wildfire. With every oversized portion and every sugary sip, waistlines expand, and so do the risks for chronic diseases like diabetes, heart disease, and even certain cancers. It's like we're all in this unhealthy race, and the finish line isn't looking so great. The statistics are the stuff of nightmares, but they're also a wake-up call. We can't keep trading long-term health for short-term satisfaction. It's time to hit the reset button and focus on what really nourishes us. After all, isn't it better to be full of life and energy rather than just... full?

Sobering Statistics:

Obesity is a significant public health concern in the U.S., with more than 2 in 5 adults (41.9%) grappling with it, and a staggering 9.2% facing severe obesity, according to the CDC. These numbers are more than just a small fry—they're a super-sized problem that demands attention.

The Standard American Diet (SAD) plays a huge role in this crisis. It's a diet heavy on sodium, light on fiber, overloaded with refined grains, and seriously lacking in fruits and veggies. Add to that a mix of sugar, saturated fats, and hydrogenated fats, and you've got a recipe for disaster. According to the CDC, approximately 50% of the calories in this diet come from carbohydrates, 15% from protein, and 35% from fat. And as we've discussed, too many carbs lead to a glucose overload, triggering insulin release, and—you guessed it—more fat storage. By cutting out gluten and refined grains to reduce inflammation and reset our metabolism, we can fuel our bodies more efficiently and give our blood sugar a much-needed break.

What is a Grain-Free Diet?

A grain-free diet involves eliminating all grains from your meals, regardless of whether they contain gluten. This means saying goodbye to foods like pasta, pizza, noodles, crackers, pancakes, bread crumbs, waffles, French toast, crepes, pastries, chips, muesli, rice cakes, breakfast cereals, cookies, and bread. Essentially, any food item that is made with grains is off the menu when following a grain-free diet. But for the purposes of this program, we're taking it a step further by also eliminating gluten—even from non-grain sources. *Why?* Because gluten has been linked to inflammation, the very thing we're trying to reduce! Gluten can trigger an immune response in some people, leading to gut irritation and inflammation, which can contribute to various health issues. By removing gluten from your diet, we aim to reduce this potential source of inflammation and help your body heal.

But again, **don't panic!** While you're kicking these grains and gluten to the curb, you'll discover that there are plenty of foods you "can" enjoy. And as you get into the swing of things, you'll find healthier versions of some of your old favorites that can easily fit into your REBOOT lifestyle— without all the gluten and refined grains dragging you down. So, let's get ready to reboot and rediscover food that loves you back!

Grain-Free Guidelines:

REMOVE:

- All gluten-containing grains: wheat & its relatives (durum, semolina, farina, farro, graham, KAMUT, einkorn, spelt, and wheat berries), rye, barley, and triticale.
- Non-gluten grains: dried corn, millet, white rice, sorghum, and oats (except sprouted oats).

INCLUDE:

- Non-grain-based flours and foods made from them: almond, flaxseed, chickpea, red lentil, sprouted oat, and coconut flours.
- Quinoa, buckwheat, and amaranth.

LIMIT:
- Starchy vegetables (1 serving per day): acorn squash, butternut squash, fresh corn, lima beans, peas, parsnips, plantain, purple cabbage, sweet potatoes, succotash, white potatoes, and yams.

INCLUDE:

- Non-starchy vegetables: artichokes, asparagus, beets, broccoli, black olives, Brussels sprouts, carrots, cauliflower, celery, green beans, leafy greens, mushrooms, onions, parsnips, peppers, salad greens, spinach, turnips, tomatoes, and zucchini.

Now that you've seen what a day in the life of eating grains and gluten looks like—complete with the rollercoaster of energy crashes and sneaky refined carbs—and now that you also know what you can and can't have on your grain and gluten-free reset, let's flip the script. What happens when someone decides to kick those refined grains and gluten to the curb? Spoiler alert: it's not all kale chips and quinoa (though they do make an appearance). Let's dive into what a typical day might look like for someone who's waving goodbye to grains and gluten and saying hello to a happier gut and more stable energy levels.

A Day in the Life of "Living Large" Without Gluten and Grains!

Morning:

You wake up feeling refreshed—no carb coma from the night before! For breakfast, you whip up some scrambled eggs with spinach and tomatoes, served with a side of avocado. Instead of the usual toast, you enjoy a slice of gluten-free, grain-free bread or some sweet potato slices lightly toasted. With a cup of green tea, you're ready to take on the day, feeling light and energized.

Mid-Morning:

When the mid-morning hunger strikes, you reach for a handful of nuts and a piece of fruit, like a crisp apple. Instead of a sugary granola bar or a pastry, you're fueling your body with nutrient-dense, whole foods that keep your energy steady.

Lunch:

For lunch, you enjoy a hearty salad with mixed greens, grilled chicken, roasted veggies, and a sprinkle of seeds for crunch. You top it off with a homemade dressing of olive oil, lemon juice, and a hint of mustard. Gone are the days of heavy sandwiches and pasta dishes that left you sluggish all afternoon. Instead, you feel satisfied but not weighed down.

Afternoon:

In the afternoon, when you need a pick-me-up, you skip the vending machine snacks and opt for some Greek yogurt with a handful of fresh berries. The protein keeps you full, and the natural sweetness of the berries satisfies your cravings.

Dinner:

Dinner is a delicious stir-fry with lean beef, broccoli, bell peppers, and zucchini, served over cauliflower rice. You season it with ginger, garlic, and tamari for a burst of flavor. No refined grains, no gluten—just a filling, nutrient-rich meal that leaves you satisfied without the bloat.

Evening:

Before bed, instead of a sugary dessert, you enjoy a warm cup of herbal tea and a small piece of dark chocolate (make sure it's gluten-free!). You go to bed feeling proud of your choices, knowing that you've nourished your body well.

Cutting out refined grains and gluten might feel like a big adjustment at first, but imagine how much clearer, lighter, and more in control of your health you will feel. As you transition, you will start to notice that those mid-afternoon energy crashes become a thing of the past, and post-meal bloating? Say goodbye to that too. By making this change, you are setting yourself up to experience more consistent energy levels and a body that feels less sluggish and more vibrant. You'll soon see that trading in those refined grains and gluten for healthier options is one of the best decisions you've made for your well-being!

Days 13-21: The Caffeine RESET

Caffeine and You: A Love Story (But Leave Out the Sugar and Creamer!)

When my kids were little, they would ask, "*Mom, have you had your coffee yet?*" It's funny now, but they knew better than to make any requests before I got my caffeine fix! Apparently, I'm not alone! The FDA says about 80% of U.S. adults consume some form of caffeine every day. Most of us rely on that morning cup of coffee or tea to kickstart the day, but caffeine is more than just a wake-up call—it's a central nervous system stimulant that affects your body in all sorts of ways.

Caffeine can be your best friend, giving you that much-needed boost, as long as you keep it within the recommended limits. According to the Mayo Clinic, most healthy adults can safely enjoy up to 400 milligrams of caffeine a day—that's roughly four 8-ounce cups of coffee. But here's the kicker: the benefits of caffeine only stick around when you don't overdo it.

Now, you might be wondering, "What's caffeine got to do with weight gain?" Well, it turns out that when you're tired, stressed, or just need a pick-me-up, that cup of joe can increase your body's cortisol levels. Cortisol, known as the "stress hormone," is produced by the adrenal glands and regulated by your brain. It's involved in everything from blood sugar regulation to controlling your sleep-wake cycle. But too much cortisol can kick your fat and carb metabolism into overdrive, leading to a surge of energy followed by an increased appetite. The result? Weight gain, especially around the midsection, which we all know is the last place we want it. You might also experience irritability, difficulty concentrating, and even high blood sugar and blood pressure.

If you're thinking about cutting back on caffeine, it's best to do it gradually. Going cold turkey could lead to withdrawal symptoms like headaches, fatigue, anxiety, and the dreaded "crankies." To make it easier, slowly reduce your intake, opt for lower-caffeine drinks, stay hydrated, get enough sleep, and add some exercise and stress reduction to your routine.

And one last thing—if you're serious about that caffeine fix, ditch the sugar and creamer. Your waistline and taste buds will thank you!

Caffeine Reset Guidelines:

- Gradually reduce and eliminate caffeine for the remainder of the REBOOT.
- Include only "organic" decaf if you are switching to decaf! This is important because chemicals are often used to reduce caffeine, which can add to our "toxic load."
- Stay hydrated.

Days 16-21: The Dairy RESET

It's time for a dairy break! During this RESET, we're putting a pause on all dairy products. That means no cow, goat, buffalo, sheep, or even camel milk (though, let's be honest, camel milk probably isn't a regular on your grocery list).

This dairy-free zone includes regular and lactose-free milk, yogurt, cheese, kefir, ice cream, butter, ghee, cream, sour cream, cream cheese, and anything containing whey or casein.

Now, don't get me wrong—dairy can be a nutritional powerhouse, offering a solid dose of calcium, vitamin D, and protein, all crucial for bone health, muscle function, and overall wellness. But for the purposes of the RESET, we're giving dairy a little vacation. Why, you ask? Well, sometimes even the best things in life need a break, and your body might just thank you for it!

While we're taking this dairy hiatus, let's take the opportunity to deepen our knowledge about dairy products, explore some exciting alternatives, and understand why this temporary break might be just what the doctor ordered. This isn't just about cutting out food; it's about gaining insights into what we consume and how it impacts our health. By exploring the role of dairy in our diet alongside discovering alternative options, we can better appreciate its benefits and potential drawbacks. This knowledge will empower you to make informed choices about reintroducing dairy later or perhaps embracing new, healthier habits. So, let's dive into some fascinating dairy facts, uncover some great alternatives, and see why giving dairy a rest might be a game-changer for your well-being!

Why is dairy such a big deal?

Well, dairy products are what we call "nutrient-dense" foods—they pack a punch with protein, calcium, B vitamins, vitamin D, and a whole bunch of other good stuff like phosphorus, potassium, and magnesium. Plus, they're one of the few foods that give you all three macronutrients: fat, carbs, and protein. Another key player in dairy is lactose, the natural sugar found in milk from mammals. Lactose isn't just there for sweetness; it provides energy and helps grow the good bacteria in your gut, which is a win for your gut health.

But let's talk fat. Milk does contain saturated fat, but the kind found in dairy might not be as bad for your heart as the saturated fat in meat. Why? It's all about the fatty acid profiles. Dairy fats are packed with more short- and medium-chain triglycerides (MCTs), which are easier for your body to use as quick energy and might even help with weight loss.

Now, the quality of these fats depends on how the animals are raised. For example, milk from grass-fed cows has up to 92% more omega-3 fatty acids and 94% more conjugated linoleic acid (CLA) than milk from conventionally raised cows. Omega-3s are superstars for hormone production, blood clotting, and keeping inflammation in check, while CLA has been linked to weight loss. So, when it comes to dairy, quality matters!

What's the Deal with Full-Fat Milk?

For years, the mantra from doctors and nutritionists was loud and clear: low-fat diets were the key to preventing heart disease. During this low-fat craze, manufacturers rolled out low-fat, fat-free, and skim dairy products as the "healthier" options, touting them as the heroes of heart health.

But here's the catch—when you strip the fat out of milk, you also strip away a lot of its nutritional goodness. To make up for the lack of flavor, these low-fat versions often got a makeover with added sugars and inflammatory vegetable oils. The problem? Those highly processed oils can cause inflammation, and even small amounts of added sugar can mess with your weight, blood sugar, and heart health. No wonder the low-fat/fat-free fad didn't exactly deliver on its promises!

Now, let's talk about full-fat dairy. Yes, it contains saturated fat, which can bump up your LDL (the "bad" cholesterol). But full-fat dairy is also packed with nutrients, and some of those saturated fats can actually lower triglycerides and boost HDL (the "good" cholesterol). In fact, a 22-year study published in *The American Journal of Clinical Nutrition* found that saturated fats might actually help protect against heart disease and stroke rather than increase the risk. But before you go on a full-fat dairy binge, remember: moderation is key! This isn't a green light to guzzle whole milk by the gallon. So, go ahead and enjoy your full-fat dairy, but keep it balanced. Follow the American Heart Association's guidelines on saturated fat, and you'll be on the right track.

Are Dairy Products Inflammatory?

Dairy can indeed stir up inflammation, but only if you have an allergy or intolerance to it. In those cases, your body reacts like it's under attack, sending out chemical messengers—think of them as tiny bodyguards like histamines, prostaglandins, and peptides. These guys rush in to heal and repair, but if they don't get the "all clear" after 72 hours, they can overstay their welcome and turn that helpful inflammation into a chronic problem.

Now, dairy isn't inflammatory for everyone. Often, people don't realize it's the culprit behind their bloating or other pesky symptoms until they cut it out and suddenly feel like a million bucks. So, if you're feeling a bit off, it might be worth considering if dairy is behind it. But remember, not everyone needs to break up with cheese—just those whose bodies are throwing up the red flags!

Organic vs. Conventional Milk: What's Really in Your Glass?

So, what's the deal with organic vs. conventional milk? Let's break it down. On conventional dairy farms, cows often get a dose of antibiotics, which can end up in the milk you pour over your cereal. The FDA says these antibiotic levels are "safe," but organic milk follows stricter rules. According to USDA guidelines, organic dairy farmers can't use antibiotics on their cows, period.

Now, you do the math:
less intervention equals less risk of those drug residues showing up in your milk.

But wait, there's more! The FDA also allows certain levels of drug residues in conventional milk, which can include antibiotics or growth hormones. Organic farms? They ban these drugs entirely. In fact, a study published in "Public Health Nutrition" (Public Health Nutr. 2019 Nov; 22(16): 2972–2980) found that organic milk had undetectable levels of antibiotics and pesticides—their milk was cleaner than a whistle!

And let's talk hormones. Cows naturally produce a growth hormone called bST to regulate milk production. Many conventional farms give cows a synthetic version of this hormone to boost milk output and cut costs. The FDA says it's safe for humans, but organic standards say "no thanks" to any synthetic hormones.

So, whether you're pouring yourself a glass or splashing it into your coffee, organic milk seems to have a bit less baggage. It's all about how much extra you want floating around in your glass!

"Udderly Delicious Alternatives: Moo-ve Over, Cow's Milk!"
(Yes, it's a bad joke, but it's also a great way to introduce some tasty milk substitutes!)

- **Hemp milk**, made from the seeds of the "Cannabis sativa" plant, offers more healthy fats and proteins than many other plant-based milks. It's also easy to digest and virtually carb-free, unless sweetened.
- **Oat milk** is higher in carbohydrates but brings the benefit of extra fiber; just be cautious, as not all oat milks are gluten-free, so reading labels is essential if you're avoiding gluten.

- **Almond milk** provides a good source of vitamin E and is low in protein, though it's not suitable for those with nut allergies. Many almond milk brands are fortified with calcium, vitamins A and D, and are naturally lower in carbs unless sweetened—unsweetened vanilla almond milk is a popular choice!

- **Coconut milk** is a safe option for those with tree nut allergies. It has less protein than almond milk but is often fortified with nutrients and contains MCTs, which may help increase HDL (good) cholesterol. Additionally, coconut kefir, a fermented coconut water with kefir grains, provides gut-friendly bacteria and is both gluten-free and dairy-free.

- **Soy milk** is nutritionally closest to cow's milk, and is higher in protein than many other alternatives. Opt for organic soy milk to ensure it's made from non-GMO soybeans and is free from conventional pesticides and herbicides.

So, as we press pause on dairy, keep these facts in mind and remember that this break is all about giving your body the best possible chance to RESET and recharge. When the time is right, you can decide if dairy deserves a comeback in your life, or if you've found new favorites that leave you feeling just as great!

As always, if you're unsure whether you can tolerate any of these alternatives, speak with your healthcare provider first to ensure they're right for you.

Dairy Reset Guidelines:

- REMOVE all dairy products, including milk, cheese, butter, kefir, and yogurt.

- INCLUDE milk alternatives such as hemp milk, almond milk, oat milk, coconut milk, and soy milk (organic).

- SUBSTITUTE conventional butter with organic coconut oil, pastured ghee, organic cold-pressed olive oil, and/or avocado oil.

- INCLUDE dairy-free yogurts (watch for added sugar content).

- INCLUDE foods labeled "VEGAN," such as plant-based cheeses and nutritional yeast.

Days 19-21: The Toxin RESET

Are You Ready To Clean Up Your Health?

The objectives of this reset are to raise your awareness about toxins, reduce your exposure to them, and remove those pesky estrogen-disrupting, thyroid-tampering, and metabolism-blocking chemicals that might be sabotaging your health and waistline.

Toxin Exposure

According to the Environmental Working Group (EWG), the average woman uses 12 personal care products each day, exposing herself to a whopping 168 unique chemicals. Men aren't entirely off the hook either, averaging five or six products a day, with teens often using even more! To make matters worse, one in 13 women is exposed to known or suspected carcinogens daily, compared to one in 23 men. So, the more products you use, the greater your chemical cocktail.

And remember, your skin is like a sponge—the largest organ in your body—and everything you slather, spray, or rub on it eventually makes its way inside. Yes, that moisturizer is doing more than just making your skin glow.

But it's not just what you put on your body. We're bombarded by toxins from all sides, including herbicides, GMOs, pesticides, and synthetic hormones lurking in our food. Over time, these toxins can build up in your bones and fat tissues, leading to a host of health concerns like eczema, diabetes, obesity, arthritis, digestive disorders, and even depression. Not exactly the kind of baggage you want to carry around.

Early symptoms of toxin overload can include unusual weight changes, brain fog or cognitive issues, sleep troubles like insomnia, mood swings or unstable behavior (hello, rollercoaster emotions!), persistent headaches, that "not-so-fresh" body odor, constipation, random body aches, and stubborn skin problems that just won't quit. So, let's get serious about this toxin reset, but remember to keep a sense of humor —after all, laughter is one of the best detoxifiers around!

Toxins and the Endocrine System: The Hormone Hijackers

Your endocrine system is like the body's control center, a network of glands and organs that uses hormones to keep everything running smoothly—from your metabolism and growth to your mood, fertility, sleep, and even blood pressure. It's a well-oiled machine... until the hormone hijackers, aka "Endocrine Disrupting Chemicals" (EDCs), come into play.

These sneaky chemicals, found in everyday items like plastic bottles, metal food cans, flame retardants, food, toys, cosmetics, and pesticides, can mimic or mess with your hormones, throwing your body's natural balance out of whack. According to the Endocrine Society, EDCs can interfere with hormone production, transportation, and metabolism, leading to a whole host of problems.

Possible Health Impacts of EDCs:

- Sperm quality and fertility issues (not exactly what you want)
- Weird changes in sex organs (no thanks)
- Endometriosis
- Early puberty (before you're ready to deal with it)
- Nervous system function getting all scrambled

- An immune system that's not quite up to the task
- Certain cancers (yikes!)
- Breathing troubles
- Metabolic issues (cue the weight gain)
- Diabetes
- Obesity
- Heart problems
- Growth issues
- Neurological and learning disabilities
- Thyroid issues that mess with your metabolism

So, How Do We "Detox" These Nasty Toxins?

Here's the good news: your body is already a detoxing pro! Your liver, kidneys, digestive system, skin, and lungs are all working around the clock to flush out toxins. While there's no solid science behind those fancy detox diets, there are plenty of ways to support your body's natural detoxification processes.

And hey, when life hands you endocrine disruptors, remember, you've got a built-in detox team on the job. Keep things balanced, stay informed, and maybe give that plastic bottle the side-eye next time!

DETOX Reset Guidelines:

- Limit alcohol consumption, as alcohol reduces your liver's ability to carry out detoxification functions.

- Aim for 7-9 hours of sleep per night, as sleep allows your brain to rest, recharge, and eliminate toxins.

- Drink plenty of water, as adequate hydration is necessary for waste removal. Reduce added sugars and processed foods, as they can lead to obesity and diabetes, which can harm your liver and kidneys.

- Consume anti-inflammatory foods, which help reduce damage caused by free radicals and, in turn, lower the risk of diseases that can impact detoxification.

- Include foods high in prebiotics and probiotics, as these keep your digestive system healthy, aid in immune function, and support proper detoxification.

- Lower your salt intake, as too much salt can increase water retention. Dehydration can affect regular bowel movements, which are essential for eliminating toxins.

- Stay active, as physical activity lowers inflammation, allows your body to work more efficiently, and enhances the detoxification process.

- READ LABELS to Avoid EDCs in Common Beauty Products.

Labels Don't Lie: The One Thing You "Must" Do to Keep Toxins at Bay

When it comes to avoiding endocrine-disrupting chemicals (EDCs) in your beauty products, reading labels is your first line of defense. Keep an eye out for some key offenders: parabens, phthalates, and sodium lauryl sulfate.

- Parabens, which are synthetic estrogen preservatives, are often found in lotions, lipsticks, and other beauty products, so opting for paraben-free options is a smart move.

- Phthalates, another synthetic estrogen, commonly show up in shampoos, deodorants, body washes, hair gels, hair sprays, and nail polishes, so check those labels and choose phthalate-free products when you can. And one more thing —avoid microwaving food in plastic containers to minimize exposure to these nasties.

- Sodium lauryl sulfate, found in toothpastes and shampoos, is another ingredient you'll want to dodge.

To make life easier, use the Environmental Working Group's [Skin Deep Database](http://www.ewg.org) to check the safety of your beauty products and find sodium lauryl sulfate-free options.

Reducing your exposure to hormone-disrupting chemicals doesn't have to be complicated. It's all about making informed choices with the products you use every day. Here are a few more tips to keep you on track:

First, ditch plastics labeled "PC" (polycarbonate) or with the recycling label #7, and never microwave food in plastic containers—unless you enjoy a side of harmful chemicals with your meal! Canned foods might be convenient, but heating food in cans can introduce unwanted toxins into your diet, so it's better to avoid them.

To stay ahead of the game, check out the Environmental Working Group's BPA product list and explore their Food Scores for healthier alternatives. And remember, fiber is your friend! Aim for at least 25 grams of fiber each day to aid digestion and help your body eliminate metabolic blockers. Finally, make regular outdoor exercise a part of your routine, and consider using a HEPA filter indoors to keep your air as clean as your conscience. By following these simple steps, you'll be well on your way to reducing your exposure to those pesky hormone-disrupting chemicals and taking control of your health.

Bottom Line...

If you're serious about reducing toxin exposure and boosting your health, stick to the basics: exercise, cut out sugar and refined carbs, spend more time outside, eat clean and hormone-free proteins, read labels, and load up on anti-inflammatory fruits and veggies.

Remember, education is key. While we might not be able to eliminate every toxin overnight (or even in 30 days), being more mindful of the products we use and the food we eat can gradually reduce our toxin load and give our metabolism the boost it deserves. So, read those labels, be picky with your products, and take it one step at a time toward a healthier you! Small changes add up, and before you know it, you'll be well on your way to feeling better, stronger, and more energized. Keep it simple, stay informed, and make choices that truly support your well-being. Your body—and your future self, will thank you!

CHAPTER 5: Optimize Your Health with Balanced Nutrition and Key Supplements
REFUEL

Congratulations on Completing the RESET! You have officially leveled up in your wellness journey—now, it's time to REFUEL and keep the momentum going! By now, you've probably realized that achieving the healthy body you "DESERVE" isn't about magic formulas, pills, shots, or quick-fix diets. It's about gaining knowledge and taking consistent steps that, over time, lead to a major transformation of your mind, body, and soul. The hard work you have put in so far has laid the foundation, and now it's time to focus on REFUELING your body with optimal nutrition—creating a lifelong eating pattern that's tailored just for you.

The following steps will help guide you in building that sustainable, personalized approach to nutrition, ensuring that the progress you've made continues to thrive as part of your everyday life. You're not just fueling your body, you are setting the stage for long-term health and happiness! With all your new knowledge and experience, you can now take control of your well-being, creating a balanced lifestyle that works uniquely for you. It's time to take what you've learned and use it to build a healthier, more vibrant future. You've got this!

Step #1: Reintroduce with Awareness- Rediscover Foods Mindfully

As you embark on Step #1 of reintroducing the foods you eliminated during the RESET, it's important to approach this process with patience and mindfulness. Over the next two weeks, you'll start reintroducing foods one by one, but don't rush—it's essential to reintroduce them in the same order you removed them, giving each food or food group 2-3 days before adding another. This deliberate pace will help you clearly see how each food affects your body, mood, and weight.

Use your journal to track your reactions as you reintroduce each food; you might discover that some foods no longer serve your body well, and that's perfectly okay. This phase is not about deprivation—it's about discovery. By carefully monitoring how your body responds, you can make informed decisions about what to keep in your diet and what to leave behind.

Remember to avoid reverting to old habits during this time. Instead, use it as an opportunity to solidify healthier alternatives and make lasting, positive changes. So take it slow, listen to your body, and enjoy the process of finding the foods that truly fuel your best self. You've got this!

Step #2: Design Your Anti-Inflammatory Plan- Build Your Personalized Eating Plan

Now that you've nailed the RESET, it's time to put what you have learned into action. The general guidelines in this section provide a summary of the essential RESET principles to help you create sustainable, tailored meals and an eating plan that suits your tastes, budget, and lifestyle. Think of it as crafting your own personalized recipe for success—but instead of just following a generic diet plan, you are curating the best ingredients to truly nourish "YOUR" body.

As you embark on this next phase, remember that you can always refer back to the full RESET guidelines whenever you need a refresher. These guidelines are here to support you, but don't hesitate to adapt them to suit your unique needs. By putting these steps into practice, you'll be creating a plan that's just right for you! So, grab your apron, and let's start crafting a delicious, healthy lifestyle that's built to last.

A. Always Choose Quality

Aim for the best quality foods and supplements you can afford because your body deserves it. Keep an eye on added sugars, limiting them to 25 grams per day for women and 36 grams for men—don't let your sweet tooth rule the day! Also, make fiber your friend by consuming 25-35 grams daily; your digestive system will thank you.

B. Build Your Balanced Plate

Fill your plate with 4-5 servings of organic (when possible) vegetables every day—spinach, kale, and broccoli should be your go-to greens. Enjoy 2-3 servings of organic fruits like berries, grapes, and plums. For carbs, opt for low-glycemic options such as quinoa, lentils, sweet potatoes, and gluten-free oats to keep your energy steady. And when it comes to protein, choose pastured eggs and poultry like chicken, duck, and turkey—quality matters!

C. Culinary Creativity with Spices

Spice up your meals with organic herbs and spices like turmeric, garlic, rosemary, and cinnamon. They're not just for flavor; they're little bursts of health!

D. Delicious, Healthy Fats

Incorporate avocados, olives, fatty fish, nuts, seeds, and cold-pressed oils like olive and avocado oil into your diet. A little healthy fat goes a long way! Don't forget to include organic bone broth, which is like liquid gold for your joints and gut. If you're into dairy, opt for organic, grass-fed full-fat dairy in moderation—a little goes a long way.

E. Extras for Gut Health

Balance your gut with prebiotics like garlic, onions, and oats, and probiotic-rich foods like yogurt, kimchi, and sauerkraut. Your gut will be your new best friend!

F. Fluid Focus

Stay hydrated by drinking plenty of filtered water. It's the simplest and most effective thing you can do for your health.

G. Go Moderate with Alcohol and Red Meat

When it comes to alcohol, limit yourself to one drink per day for women and up to two for men, choosing low-sugar options like dry wines or clear spirits with sugar-free mixers. For red meat, enjoy it 1-2 times per week, choosing lean, grass-fed cuts and pairing them with lots of veggies.

H. Healthy Brews

Enjoy your coffee or tea, but keep it under 400 mg of caffeine per day—because life is always better with a little caffeine. If you're choosing decaf coffee, always opt for organic to limit unwanted chemicals.

I. Informed Seafood Selections

Choose wild-caught seafood and low-mercury fish like salmon, trout, sardines, and shrimp. Always check for the latest guidelines to keep it safe.

By following these steps, you're not just creating an eating plan—you're laying the foundation for a lifetime of health and vitality. Keep it up—you're doing amazing!

Step #3: Cleanse Your Environment- Minimize Toxins, Maximize Health

Reducing your toxic load is simpler than it might seem! Here are some straightforward tips to help you minimize exposure to harmful chemicals and keep your body in top shape:

First, choose organic whenever possible—whether it's produce, meats, or dairy. By doing this, you'll cut down on your intake of pesticides, hormones, and antibiotics, giving your body a much-needed break from the chemical overload. Next, make sure to wash your fruits and vegetables thoroughly. Using a natural produce wash or soaking them in a water and vinegar mix can help remove pesticides—because who really wants a side of chemicals with their salad?

Avoiding processed foods is also key. These are like the drama queens of the food world, bringing unnecessary artificial additives, preservatives, and unhealthy fats to the party. Sticking to whole foods is a safer bet for a drama-free meal. Another simple switch is to use glass or stainless steel containers instead of plastic for storing food. It's a small change, but one that helps you avoid BPA and other toxins. Your future self—and the planet—will thank you!

Filtering your water is another easy step. Think of it as giving your tap water a spa day, resulting in clean, safe water without added contaminants. When it comes to canned foods, it's best to limit them since they can sneak in BPA through their linings. Fresh or frozen options are healthier, or look for cans labeled BPA-free.

Being mindful of fish consumption is also important. Opt for wild-caught seafood and fish that are low in mercury, like salmon, sardines, and trout. For more detailed advice, check out the Environmental Working Group's guidelines—because no one needs extra heavy metals in their diet.

Finally, ditch the non-stick cookware and go for stainless steel, cast iron, or ceramic options instead. Your omelet might stick a little, but at least it won't come with a side of questionable chemicals.

By making these informed choices and adapting the guidelines to fit your lifestyle, you're taking charge of your health and becoming your own health advocate. With the knowledge you've gained throughout the REBOOT, you're not just a passive participant—you're actively shaping your own health journey. Use your newfound understanding to make decisions that support your well-being, and don't hesitate to stand up for what's best for your body. After all, no one knows your health better than you do!

Step#4: Assess Your Nutrient Needs- Supplement Wisely, Thrive Fully

We know that chronic inflammation can pave the way for diseases like type 2 diabetes, heart disease, obesity, and autoimmune disorders. After completing the REBOOT, you will have learned that anti-inflammatory foods, stress management, adequate sleep, and exercise can help combat chronic inflammation. But did you know that certain supplements can also offer a bit of extra support?

First things first... the backbone of your anti-inflammatory diet should be high-quality, nutrient-dense, organic (when possible), whole foods.

However, sometimes, even the best diet needs a little help. Modern agricultural methods have left our soil nutrient-deficient, stress and chronic disease can increase our nutritional needs, and let's not forget about the extra toxins we encounter daily or that time we skipped a workout. All of these factors can make it challenging to meet our nutritional requirements without some supplemental help.

That said, it's crucial to understand that no supplement can magically fix a poor diet. Supplements are not a replacement for the enzymes and nutritional compounds found in real food. Therefore, it's essential to work with a qualified health professional to determine your unique nutrient needs and help you identify high quality supplements in the right amounts for your specific health goals.

Choosing the right supplement is critical! Unfortunately, the market is flooded with sub-standard products full of fillers, synthetic nutrients, and preservatives that can do more harm than good.

When shopping for supplements, it's crucial to prioritize quality and safety. Start by purchasing supplements from reputable manufacturers that follow certified Good Manufacturing Practices (cGMP), ensuring they meet FDA standards and undergo third-party testing for quality assurance. Next, always consult with a Registered Dietitian or your healthcare provider to determine your specific nutritional needs. This step is vital to avoid unnecessary or incorrect supplementation. Finally, stick to the dosage instructions provided on the packaging unless your healthcare professional advises otherwise. These steps will help you make informed decisions and safely incorporate supplements into your routine.

Remember, supplements should complement a healthy diet, not replace it. When in doubt, seek professional advice—self-prescribing supplements can be risky, and getting it right is crucial for your health!

Nutrients That May Play a Role in Reducing Inflammation...

Let's talk about some of the key players in the fight against inflammation. But before we dive in, let me be clear—I'm "NOT" telling you to load up on all these supplements like it's a Black Friday sale. It's crucial to determine if you're actually deficient in any of these nutrients first, and work with a Registered Dietitian or your healthcare provider to figure out what "YOU" specifically need. Trust me, when it comes to supplements, more is not always better.

B Vitamins

B Vitamins are like the Swiss Army knife of your body—versatile and essential for everything from energy production to maintaining a healthy nervous system. Vitamin B6, in particular, is a rockstar when it comes to fighting inflammation. A deficiency in B6 has been linked to higher levels of inflammation markers like C-Reactive Protein. Also, if you're low in B6, B9 (folate), or B12, you might see elevated levels of homocysteine—a risk factor for heart disease and rheumatoid arthritis. Foods like fish, beef liver, leafy greens, and nuts are good sources, or consider a quality B Complex supplement.

Vitamin C

Vitamin C isn't just for preventing scurvy—it's a powerful antioxidant that helps protect cells from damage and supports important processes in your body, like collagen production and neurotransmitter creation. The body absorbs vitamin C best when taken in amounts of about 200 to 500 milligrams at a time. How well your body absorbs it can depend on factors like the type of vitamin C you are taking, whether you are also getting other nutrients that help with absorption, and your overall health. Foods rich in vitamin C include berries, citrus fruits, tomatoes, and vegetables like broccoli. The recommended daily amount is 90 mg for men and 75 mg for women. Just be cautious—taking more than 2000 mg a day can lead to some uncomfortable stomach issues.

Vitamin D3

Vitamin D3 is a fat-soluble nutrient that's crucial for immune health, and a deficiency can crank up your inflammation levels. While your body can make Vitamin D from sunlight, it's not always reliable due to factors like sunscreen use, skin type, and living in areas with less sun exposure. The daily value is 800 IU (20 mcg), but adults should generally stick to no more than 4000 IU per day unless otherwise advised. You can find Vitamin D in foods like oily fish, egg yolks, and beef liver, but definitely check your levels with a healthcare provider before supplementing.

Garlic

Garlic isn't just for warding off vampires; it's loaded with anti-inflammatory compounds, especially a sulfur compound called allicin. This pungent little bulb has antiviral, antifungal, and antibacterial properties too. For maximum benefit, raw garlic is your best bet—cooking can reduce its allicin content. But a word of caution: too much raw garlic can irritate the digestive tract, and if you're on blood thinners, you might want to keep it in check. A clove or two a day should do the trick.

Ginger

Ginger has been spicing up kitchens and medicine cabinets for centuries. It's a potent anti-inflammatory thanks to compounds like gingerol and zingerone. These compounds may help reduce inflammation in conditions like cardiovascular disease and arthritis. But remember, moderation is key—too much ginger can mess with certain medications, like blood thinners, so check with your doctor or dietitian first.

Green Tea Extract

Green tea is rich in polyphenols, including EGCG, which packs a serious anti-inflammatory punch. Studies show green tea may help with everything from lowering LDL cholesterol to boosting metabolism. A few (organic) cups a day (3-5) should suffice, but the optimal amount can vary depending on your individual health needs. As always, consult with your healthcare provider.

Turmeric (Curcumin)

Turmeric's curcumin is a powerful anti-inflammatory and antioxidant. It's been shown to help reduce inflammation in conditions like heart disease, diabetes, and some cancers. But curcumin alone isn't easily absorbed—pair it with piperine (found in black pepper) and a healthy fat to increase its bioavailability by up to 2000%.

Omega-3 Fatty Acids

Omega-3s are essential for heart health and reducing inflammation. These fats are vital for your body's well-being and can be found in fatty fish like salmon, mackerel, and sardines, as well as in plant-based sources like flaxseeds and chia seeds. The American Heart Association recommends that individuals with heart disease consume about 1 gram of EPA and DHA per day, preferably from food sources. While supplements can help fill in the gaps, it's best to meet your omega-3 needs through diet whenever possible. Omega-3 supplements can interact with certain medications, such as blood thinners, so it's crucial to consult a healthcare professional or a Registered Dietitian before starting any supplement regimen. This ensures that you're getting the right amount without risking any adverse effects.

Bottom Line...supplements can be a helpful addition to a well-rounded diet, but they are not a cure-all. Always choose quality products from reputable manufacturers and work with a healthcare provider to tailor them to your needs. Always remember, food first—there's no replacement for a balanced, nutrient-rich diet!

Congratulations on completing the REFUEL phase of your REBOOT!

By now, you've not only RESET your metabolism but also learned how to REFUEL your body with the optimal nutrition it needs to thrive. You have discovered how to nourish yourself with foods that support your unique needs, reduce inflammation, improve gut health, and promote overall well-being. But remember, the journey doesn't stop here.

If you're the type of person who's curious about tailoring your nutrition even further—like figuring out exactly how many carbs you need or how much protein is right for you—then you will want to keep going. In Chapter 7, I will introduce you to Phil's 30 Day REBOOT online course, where we will dive deeper into your specific nutritional needs. This course will guide you through the process of calculating your ideal macronutrient ratios, setting personalized goals, and continuing to refine your healthy lifestyle. So, if you're ready to satisfy that curiosity and take your health to the next level, stay tuned!

Next, we're diving into the REWIRE phase—where we focus on the mind-body connection and solidifying the habits that will sustain your health long-term. The REWIRE process is all about rewiring your mindset, behaviors, and routines to ensure that the positive changes you've made stick. This is where we shift from simply following a plan to fully embracing a new lifestyle that supports your healthiest, happiest self. Let's get ready to rewire your thinking, enhance your self-care, and truly transform your relationship with food and health!

CHAPTER 6: It's Time for Some Serious Self-Care
The REWIRE

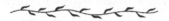

So, you've nailed the RESET, powered through REFUEL, and now you're probably feeling pretty fantastic. But there's one more crucial piece of this wellness puzzle we need to talk about—self-care. And no, I'm not just talking about the occasional bubble bath or face mask (though those are fabulous too). We're diving into the heavy hitters: exercise and movement, sleep, and stress management. These are the pillars that hold up the entire REBOOT structure, and let's be honest, they're often the first things we toss aside when life gets chaotic.

Think of these habits as the secret sauce that makes all your hard work stick. They're the glue that keeps your newfound healthy lifestyle from falling apart. So, let's get into the nitty-gritty of how to move more, sleep better, and keep your stress levels in check—because trust me, your body will thank you, and you might even find yourself smiling more along the way. After all, a little humor and a lot of self-care go a long way!

When it comes to achieving better health, we often zero in on the usual suspects: poor nutrition, lack of exercise, smoking, and indulging in one too many cocktails. But here's the thing—your mind and body are like best friends; they're deeply connected. Focusing solely on physical health without addressing your emotional well-being is like trying to bake a cake without flour. Sure, you might get something resembling a cake, but it won't be nearly as satisfying. To create new, healthier habits, you need a holistic approach that balances both physical and emotional wellness.

As you work to improve your physical health, it's just as crucial to nurture your mental and emotional state. Making significant changes in multiple areas of your life doesn't happen overnight, so give yourself time and, more importantly, grace during the process. This section of the REBOOT will help you REWIRE your brain, forming new, healthier habits that stick. It's not just about what you do; it's about how you think and feel about these changes, creating a lasting impact on your overall well-being.

Forming new habits isn't as simple as sticking with them for a few weeks. While the old "21-day rule" suggested by Dr. Maxwell Maltz might have worked for some, more recent research from the NIH reveals that it can actually take anywhere from 18 to 254 days to establish a new habit, with an average of 66 days before it becomes automatic. The timeline varies for each person, but the key to success is consistency and patience as you develop these life-enhancing habits.

There's no one-size-fits-all approach, so the only timeline that truly matters is the one that works for you. To help yourself along the way, consider recruiting your people—friends, family, and healthcare providers—for support. Partnering up with someone can make the journey more enjoyable, as teamwork makes the dream work. Practice the REBOOT motto: Progress Over Perfection! Perfection is overrated, so focus on your progress, no matter how small. Track your results and be kind to yourself—celebrate the wins, no matter how small they may seem.

With these steps in mind, you're well on your way to rewiring your brain and embracing a healthier, happier you! Now, let's dive into how exercise, sleep, and stress management can further support you on this amazing journey.

Exercise and Movement

Remember when you were a kid, running around outside, laughing, skipping, and jumping without a care in the world? That was pure joy—joy through movement! So where did that joyous feeling go? As we grow up and responsibilities start piling on, exercise often gets bumped to the dreaded "to-do list" and loses its fun factor. But here's the truth: as adults, we need to bring that joy back by making exercise a habit—because it really is good for you! Let's break down why...

Exercise cranks up the production of endorphins—those magical "feel-good" hormones that boost your mood and help manage stress and anxiety. It also revs up your metabolism, making it easier to burn calories and manage your weight. Regular movement keeps your bones and muscles strong, lubricates your joints, and helps you stay flexible as you age. If you're looking for an energy boost, exercise can give you a natural lift that lasts all day. Plus, it's a powerful tool in reducing the risk of chronic diseases by improving insulin sensitivity, lowering blood pressure, and decreasing cholesterol levels.

Exercise is also a brain health booster, promoting cognitive resilience, reducing age-related brain shrinkage, and helping fend off dementia. And if better sleep sounds appealing, exercise can help you sleep more soundly and feel more energized during the day. To top it all off, exercise can even spice up your sex life—talk about a win-win!

Let's face it—exercise can improve just about every aspect of your life! According to the CDC, an estimated 110,000 deaths per year could be prevented if U.S. adults aged 40 and older added even a small amount of moderate-to-vigorous activity to their daily routines. Just 10 minutes a day could make a world of difference. So, why not bring back that joy in motion and make exercise something you actually look forward to? Your body—and your mind—will thank you!

So, what are the recommendations?

The American Heart Association recommends that adults aim for at least 150 minutes of moderate-intensity aerobic activity per week, such as brisk walking or light cycling, or 75 minutes of vigorous aerobic activity, like running or high-intensity interval training. You can mix and match these activities throughout the week to fit your schedule. Additionally, it's important to include strength training at a moderate to high intensity on at least two days per week—this could be anything from resistance exercises to lifting weights.

But don't stop there! The guidelines also emphasize the importance of sitting less. Even light activity can help counteract the negative effects of being too sedentary. For those looking to maximize their benefits, aim for 300 minutes (5 hours) of activity per week, gradually increasing the amount and intensity over time.

Now, I know these guidelines might seem daunting at first. You might be thinking, "How am I supposed to fit all this into my busy life?" But remember the REBOOT MOTTO: Progress Over Perfection! You don't have to do it all at once.

In fact, when we look at the habits of people in the "Blue Zones"—regions where individuals frequently live to 100 and beyond—what stands out is not hours spent in the gym, but rather the incorporation of natural movement into daily life. These individuals walk frequently, garden, and engage in household chores, staying active throughout the day. Their secret isn't intense workouts but consistent, moderate physical activity woven into their routines.

Supporting this idea, research from the National Institutes of Health (NIH) and the CDC in 2020 found that aiming for about 9,000 steps per day is ideal for general health, and 7,000 steps per day is optimal for cardiovascular health. So, lace up those sneakers, and start stepping! Your heart—and your future self—will thank you.

At the end of the day... JUST MOVE! Whether it's dancing with your kids, grooving in front of the mirror, walking while chatting on the phone, strolling with a friend, doing active chores, taking the stairs, or hopping on a bike—just keep moving! Your heart will be grateful.

And, of course, before starting any new exercise routine, make sure to check in with your healthcare provider to ensure it's safe for you.

Sleep

You spend about one-third of your life asleep, and while some people might think of this as a waste of time or joke, "I'll sleep when I'm dead," they don't realize just how true that saying could be—only not in the way they intended! Modern living often treats sleep as a luxury, but it's essential for good health and the optimal functioning of your brain and body. Just like exercise and good nutrition, quality sleep boosts your brain performance, mood, and overall health.

Sleep helps reduce inflammation in the body, which is linked to various chronic diseases. It also plays a key role in weight management—lack of sleep increases ghrelin (the hormone that makes you hungry) and decreases leptin (the hormone that makes you feel full), leading to overeating. Moreover, good sleep enhances your memory and cognitive performance, making you sharper during the day.
Sleep is also crucial for heart health; it regulates blood pressure, a major risk factor for heart disease, and may even strengthen your heart. Additionally, getting enough sleep can stabilize your mood by improving emotional regulation and reducing the risk of depression. Sleep also helps regulate insulin, reducing the risk of type 2 diabetes, and strengthens your immune system, making you better at fighting off illnesses. For athletes, sleep is like a natural performance enhancer, improving reaction times, endurance, and overall physical performance.

Sleep isn't just "down time." It's when your body repairs itself—it's your body's version of self-care! While you're dreaming, your brain is hard at work, clearing out waste and doing some serious maintenance. From blood vessels to the immune system, sleep is when your body gets its tune-up. Without enough sleep, these essential processes get disrupted, leading to some pretty serious health consequences. So, do yourself a favor and GO TO SLEEP—your body and mind will thank you for it!

How Much Sleep is Enough?

The American Academy of Sleep Medicine recommends that adults aim for at least seven hours of sleep per night, but for most people, the sweet spot is between seven to nine hours.

However, if you're consistently clocking in at six hours or less, you might be inviting some unwelcome guests—like inflammation—into your life, even if you consider yourself healthy. And let's face it, inflammation isn't exactly the life of the party. It can lead to metabolic issues that increase your risk of obesity, type 2 diabetes, heart disease, and dementia. Notice a pattern? Poor nutrition, lack of exercise, and now, lack of sleep—they all conspire together to wreak havoc on your health.

But it's not just about how much sleep you get; the quality matters too. If you're waking up feeling like you've been hit by a truck, chances are your sleep isn't as restful as it should be. Factors like age, mental health, sleep disorders (such as sleep apnea or restless leg syndrome), too much screen time before bed, late-night social media scrolling, a heavy meal, or that glass of wine before hitting the sack can all sabotage your sleep quality.

Here are a few tips to help you catch those elusive z's: Create a peaceful sleep environment—your bedroom should be a sanctuary. Turn off electronic devices at least one hour before bed to give your brain time to wind down. Stick to a regular sleep schedule by going to bed and waking up around the same times each day. Avoid caffeine and alcohol, especially in the four to six hours leading up to bedtime. Eat earlier, aiming to finish meals two to three hours before bed. Create a relaxing bedtime ritual like meditation or a warm bath to signal your body that it's time to sleep. Exercise during the day to tire out your body, making it easier to fall asleep. Limit daytime naps to 20 minutes or less to avoid disrupting your nighttime sleep.

Self-care isn't just about what you eat or how much you move—getting enough quality sleep is just as crucial. So do yourself a favor: turn off Netflix, stop doom-scrolling on social media, and tuck yourself in earlier. Consider sleep your body's nightly "thank you" for all that it does.

Stress Management

I can't help but laugh as I write this because, honestly, stress management should be a mandatory class for adults! Stress is a tricky beast. Not only does it mess with your emotions, but it also sneaks into your body and wreaks havoc in ways you might not even realize—until it's too late. And trust me, I learned this the hard way. I didn't manage stress well, and my immune system ended up paying the price! Stress is a natural physical and mental reaction to life's ups and downs. A little bit of stress, like acute inflammation, can actually be beneficial; it keeps you on your toes. But chronic stress? Well, that's a whole different ball game. Like chronic inflammation, prolonged stress can wear you down and seriously mess with your overall well-being.

Chronic stress can wreak havoc on your body and mind in more ways than you might realize. For starters, it can give you headaches and back pain that make it feel like you're literally carrying the weight of the world on your shoulders. It can also lead to anxiety and depression, turning your mood upside down and making you feel like you're on an emotional rollercoaster. Your gut isn't spared either—chronic stress can cause everything from nausea to diarrhea, making your digestive system feel like it's in constant turmoil.

As if that weren't enough, stress can spike your blood sugar, increasing your risk of type 2 diabetes and obesity, and it can even mess with your libido, leading to fertility issues. Chronic stress doesn't stop there; it can disrupt your sleep, leaving you feeling foggy-brained and exhausted. It also forces your heart to work overtime, raising your blood pressure and increasing your risk of a stroke or heart attack. And here's the kicker: it can weaken your immune system, making it harder for your body to fight off infections and recover from illnesses or injuries.

Chronic stress, much like chronic inflammation, is no joke. That's why it's crucial to learn how to manage stress effectively. Your ability to handle stress is influenced by various factors—genes, childhood experiences, culture, economics— you name it. While some of these factors are beyond your control, there are ways to build up your resilience and prevent stress from taking over your life. Let's explore some strategies to help you manage or reduce stress.

Stress Management Techniques

Managing stress effectively can feel like trying to juggle flaming torches, but with the right techniques, you can keep those torches in the air and avoid getting burned! Here are some stress management strategies that not only help you keep your cool but can also add a little more joy to your life:

First...get moving! Exercise isn't just about staying fit— it cranks up those feel-good hormones called endorphins. So, whether you're jogging, dancing, or even chasing your dog around the yard, make movement a priority. Speaking of dogs, spending time with your furry friends is a fantastic stress buster —they're always ready to listen, and they never judge!

Mindfulness practices like yoga and meditation can work wonders, too. Not only do they help calm your mind, but they've also been shown to reduce inflammation. And while you're at it, make sure you're getting enough sleep—because let's face it, everything seems worse when you're tired.

Cut back on the caffeine, which can make you jittery and more anxious. Instead, fuel your body with a healthy diet that supports both your physical and mental health. Building strong social connections is also key—whether it's friends, family, or a supportive online community, having people to lean on can make a world of difference.

In today's tech-heavy world, it's also important to limit your phone and screen time. Unplug, unwind, and give your mind a break. And hey, if you haven't already, check out Kim's book to figure out "Who Is Driving Your Bus." Reframing your thoughts and emotions can completely shift how you deal with stress.

Don't forget to talk to yourself kindly—positive self-talk can uplift your spirits when the going gets tough. And perhaps most importantly, learn to set boundaries and say "NO" when you need to. It's not selfish—it's self-preservation! By implementing these strategies, you'll be well on your way to taming the stress beast and enjoying a more balanced, joyful life.

Master the Art of Self-Care—"Your" Recipe for a Longer, Healthier Life

As we wrap up the REWIRE section of your REBOOT journey, it's time to reflect on the powerful habits and insights you've gained—habits that aren't just good advice, but are backed by solid research from some of the biggest names in the health field, including the NIH, CDC, and Harvard Health.

These strategies are designed to enhance your overall well-being, reduce the risk of chronic diseases, and promote longevity.

Let's start with your "eating plan" (because let's face it, we know diets don't work). By focusing on filling your plate with fruits, veggies, whole grains, and healthy fats while keeping red and processed meats, sugary drinks, and trans fats to a minimum, you are not just following some temporary trend—you're committing to a *sustainable* way of eating that truly nourishes your body. This isn't about restrictive dieting; it's about fueling your life with the best foods that support long-term health and vitality. So, forget about diets and embrace this empowering way of eating that's designed to help you thrive.

Next up, the importance of "exercise" can't be overstated. Aim for at least 3.5 hours of moderate-to-vigorous exercise each week; or you can count your steps and follow the National Institutes of Health (NIH) and the CDC's recommendation to complete 9,000 steps per day for general health, and 7,000 steps per day for optimal cardiovascular health. This could be anything from dancing around your living room to hiking or hitting the gym. The key is to keep moving because, as they say, motion is lotion for your joints and muscles!

Let's not forget the critical role of "sleep". Quality rest is vital for repairing your body and maintaining overall health. Aim for 7-9 hours of sleep each night, ensuring your body gets the downtime it needs to reset and recharge. Good sleep habits can also help reduce inflammation and support weight management.

Managing "stress" is another essential component of your REWIRE journey. Whether it's through meditation, deep breathing, or simply taking time to unwind, effective stress management is crucial for both your mental and physical health. High stress levels can wreak havoc on your body, leading to a host of health issues, like increased inflammation and poor gut health, so finding ways to manage stress effectively is key to long-term well-being.

In the REBOOT, we may not dive deeply into "smoking cessation", but it's universally understood that kicking this habit is one of the best things you can do for your health. If you're still lighting up, quitting now can drastically improve your health outcomes and extend your life.

Alcohol consumption should also be kept in check. Moderate drinking—no more than one drink a day for women and up to two for men—can fit into a healthy lifestyle, but it's important to be mindful of how much and how often you indulge.

Finally, maintaining a "healthy weight" is about more than just looking good; it's about keeping your body running smoothly for years to come. Monitoring your weight and waist size can help you avoid the risks associated with obesity, including heart disease, diabetes, and other chronic conditions.

These habits aren't just about adding years to your life— they're about adding life to your years.

Prioritizing self-care through good nutrition, regular exercise, quality sleep, and effective stress management isn't a luxury; it's a necessity for living a balanced, fulfilling life. Self-care isn't selfish—it's about ensuring you have the energy and vitality to give the world the best of you, not just what's left of you.

The impact of these habits can be profound. According to Harvard Health, if you start practicing them consistently from age 50 onward, you could add over a decade to your life. That's right—a whole decade! Women who follow these habits could live to 93, compared to just 79 for those who don't. Similarly, men could extend their lives to nearly 88, as opposed to 75. Not too shabby, right? By embracing these simple but powerful habits, you're not just adding time to your life—you're enriching every moment of it.

Remember...

You are beautiful, strong, smart, and worth every bit of the effort it takes to live your healthiest life. These qualities make you truly unstoppable.

Not only have you "CRACKED THE FOOD CODE", but by embracing self-care in all its forms—nutrition, exercise, sleep, and stress management—you've also "CRACKED THE HEALTH CODE". Remember, the commitment you're making to yourself isn't just about physical wellness; it's about honoring your worth and embracing the life you deserve. Every step you take, every healthy choice you make, reinforces the fact that you are deserving of all the health, happiness, and vitality that life has to offer. So keep going—you're worth it!

CHAPTER 7: The Next Step
Phil's 30-Day REBOOT

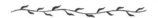

Congratulations on making it this far! You've "CRACKED THE FOOD CODE" and fully embraced the REBOOT principles, setting yourself firmly on the path to a healthier, happier you. But let's be honest—this journey is just getting started! Some of you will take the information in this book and run with it, confidently integrating what you've learned into your daily life. Others might be craving a more structured approach, eager to dive deeper into how to meet their daily nutritional needs by mastering their macros.

If you're excited to elevate your health and wellness game and need that extra bit of guidance, let me introduce you to Phil's 30-Day REBOOT—a comprehensive, structured, and supportive online program designed to give you everything you need to truly succeed. This next step isn't just a continuation; it's a powerful leap forward. Whether you're looking to fine-tune your eating plan or get a handle on your macros, this program is tailored to help you achieve your goals.

What are "macros," you ask? Macros, short for macronutrients, are like the three musketeers of your diet: carbs, protein, and fat. They each have their own superpowers —carbs for quick energy, protein for muscle building, and fat for keeping you full and fabulous. Just don't ask them to share the spotlight—they're each pretty essential!

What's in the 30-Day REBOOT?

This program is your go-to guide for resetting your health anytime you need it—whether after a holiday binge, a vacation, or simply when you feel the need to get back on track.

Here's a sneak peek at what you can expect:

- *Personalized Nutrition Guidance:* Determine your basal metabolic rate and adjust for exercise so you can understand exactly how much you need to eat to fuel your body. You will also receive guidelines on how to set your macros (carbohydrates, proteins, and fats) based on your unique health goals.

- *Comprehensive Food Tracking:* With a cutting-edge food tracking app, you can easily track your macros, added sugars, and fiber intake. You can even create custom meals and recipes to see exactly how they contribute to your daily macronutrient targets.

- *Extensive Recipe Index:* Explore a rich collection of delicious and nutritious recipes, each one thoughtfully selected to support your health journey. And there's more—this recipe index is filled with Phil's personal favorites, from quick snacks and refreshing drinks to essential ingredients that will take your meals to the next level. Plus, discover Phil's top places to shop, exclusive coupons, and direct shopping links that make meal prep effortless. Whether you're planning a full meal or grabbing a healthy snack, this index is your go-to resource for keeping your palate satisfied and your body energized.

- *Community Support:* Join our private Facebook community where you can share your journey, ask questions, and get support from others who are on the same path. There's nothing like a little encouragement to keep you going!

- *Exclusive Supplement Savings:* Unlock access to carefully selected supplement recommendations tailored to support your health journey. Plus, enjoy discounts on many of these supplements, making it easier and more affordable to stay on track with your wellness goals.

- *Add-On Coaching Options:* Need a little extra help? We offer optional coaching services to provide personalized support and guidance to help you stay on track and achieve your goals.

- *Lifetime Access*: Once you're in, you're in for life! You can revisit the program whenever you need a reset, whether it's after a vacation, a holiday season, or just because you want to refresh your healthy habits.

- *Exclusive Content:* Stay up to date with newsletters, new food products, and much more. We're constantly adding new resources to keep you informed and inspired.

Why Join the 30-Day REBOOT?

This isn't just another diet program—it's a lifestyle transformation. The 30-Day REBOOT gives you the tools and resources to make lasting changes, tailored to your individual needs. Plus, with lifetime access, you can continue to reap the benefits long after the 30 days are over. Whether you're looking to lose weight, improve your energy levels, or simply feel better in your own skin, this program has everything you need to succeed. *So, are you ready to take the plunge?* Lace up your sneakers, grab your water bottle, and let's get started! Phil's 30-Day REBOOT is waiting for you. Let's make this your healthiest year yet! To get started, visit:

https://www.philknowsfood.com

"Living in a state of gratitude is the gateway to grace."
Arianna Huffington

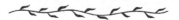

Let me begin by expressing just how deeply grateful I am for you. It takes immense courage to step up and take back control of your health, to make that bold decision to prioritize your well-being. Your commitment to this journey fills me with immense pride, and I want you to know how powerful that is.

Educating yourself to better your quality of life is no small feat. It's a reflection of your strength, resilience, and determination to make meaningful changes—one step, one choice at a time. You have not only completed your personal REBOOT, but you've also laid the foundation for a healthier lifestyle, one that can treat, reverse, and prevent chronic diseases that so many struggle with.

This program isn't just a one-time deal; it's a tool you can use again and again, anytime you need to RESET your mind, body, and soul. You have the power and the tools to take back control of your health, and that's something to be incredibly proud of.

By learning how to RESET, REFUEL, and REWIRE your brain, you have unlocked the secrets to *Cracking The Food Code*— and in doing so, you've also discovered the truth: "DIETS DON'T WORK"! You weren't crazy to think that those quick fixes and restrictive plans never led to lasting change. Instead, you've developed your own unique, sustainable eating pattern that aligns perfectly with your goals and lifestyle. This approach empowers you to take control of your health like never before, putting an end to the cycle of failed diets. No more quick fixes—just real, lasting change that honors your body and supports your long-term well-being.

But remember, this is a process. Give yourself some grace along the way. You're going to be learning and expanding your REBOOT knowledge every single day. It's important to have realistic expectations and practice PROGRESS OVER PERFECTION! Celebrate your wins, no matter how small, and know that every step forward is a step in the right direction.

Most importantly, remember that you are worthy of health, joy, and all the good things life has to offer. You deserve to feel empowered and accomplished, and to live your life with confidence in your own abilities.

It's my hope that you'll continue using the tools from this REBOOT to keep creating the healthiest version of yourself. Thank you from the bottom of my heart for allowing me to be your guide on this journey. Where you go from here is entirely up to you, but I have no doubt you're on the path to greatness!

In Health,

Philippa xo

PHILKN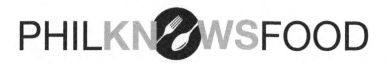WSFOOD

Cracking The Food Code
THE REBOOT GUIDE

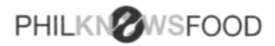

The 21 Day RESET At-A-Glance

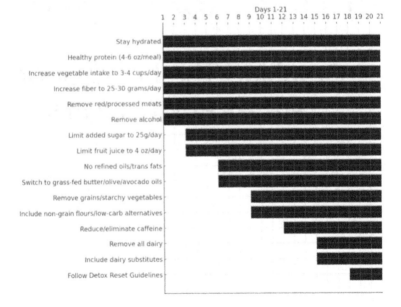

	Days 1-21
	1 2 3 4 5 6 7 8 9 10 11 12 13 14 15 16 17 18 19 20 21
Stay hydrated	
Healthy protein (4-6 oz/meal)	
Increase vegetable intake to 3-4 cups/day	
Increase fiber to 25-30 grams/day	
Remove red/processed meats	
Remove alcohol	
Limit added sugar to 25g/day	
Limit fruit juice to 4 oz/day	
No refined oils/trans fats	
Switch to grass-fed butter/olive/avocado oils	
Remove grains/starchy vegetables	
Include non-grain flours/low-carb alternatives	
Reduce/eliminate caffeine	
Remove all dairy	
Include dairy substitutes	
Follow Detox Reset Guidelines	

Anti-Inflammatory Pantry Staples
Low in Sugar & Gluten Free

This pantry list includes a variety of staples that will help you create delicious and nutritious meals while following an anti-inflammatory meal plan that is low in sugar and gluten-free.

Whole Grains and Legumes
- Quinoa
- Brown rice
- Gluten-free oats
- Lentils (green, red, or brown)
- Chickpeas (canned or dried)
- Black beans
- Buckwheat
- Millet

Health Fats and Oils
- Extra virgin olive oil
- Avocado oil
- Flaxseed oil
- Coconut oil (for occasional use)
- Olives: black, green, kalamata
- Nuts: almonds, walnuts, cashews, pistachios
- Seeds: chia seeds, flaxseeds, sunflower seeds, pumpkin seeds
- Nut butters: almond butter, cashew butter

Proteins
- Canned tuna or salmon (low in mercury)
- Canned sardines
- Dried or canned beans (chickpeas, black beans, etc.)
- Canned or jarred wild-caught fish
- Organic or pasture-raised eggs

- Smoked salmon (lox)
- Turkey bacon (uncured, nitrate-free)
- Grass-fed meats (frozen or fresh)
- Organic, pasture-raised poultry (frozen or fresh)
- Plain Greek yogurt (full-fat, unsweetened)

Herbs, Spices and Condiments
- Dried herbs: oregano, thyme, rosemary, basil, dill
- Spices: turmeric, cumin, paprika, cinnamon, nutmeg, black pepper
- Garlic (fresh or dried)
- Onion powder
- Sea salt or Himalayan pink salt
- Peppercorns (black or mixed)
- Apple cider vinegar
- Balsamic vinegar
- Dijon mustard
- Capers
- Pesto (homemade or store-bought, gluten-free)
- Tahini

Vegetables (Fresh or Frozen)
- Leafy greens (spinach, kale, arugula)
- Broccoli
- Cauliflower
- Bell peppers
- Zucchini
- Cucumbers
- Tomatoes (fresh, canned, or sun-dried)
- Carrots
- Sweet potatoes
- Avocados
- Onions
- Garlic
- Mushrooms

- Artichokes (canned or jarred)

Fruits (Fresh or Frozen)
- Berries (blueberries, raspberries, strawberries)
- Apples
- Pears
- Grapes
- Citrus fruits (lemons, oranges, limes)
- Plums
- Cherries (fresh or dried, unsweetened)
- Figs (fresh or dried, unsweetened)
- Dates (unsweetened)

Dairy and Dairy Alternatives
- Unsweetened almond milk or coconut milk
- Feta cheese
- Goat cheese
- Parmesan cheese (for occasional use)

Snacks
- Raw nuts: almonds, walnuts, pistachios
- Seeds: pumpkin seeds, sunflower seeds
- Hummus (homemade or store-bought, gluten-free)
- Gluten-free crisp-bread or crackers
- Wilde Protein Chips (gluten-free)
- Seaweed snacks
- Dark chocolate (70% cocoa or higher, low in sugar)

Beverages
- Herbal teas: green tea, peppermint, chamomile
- Black coffee (unsweetened)
- Sparkling water (plain or with natural flavors)
- Coconut water (unsweetened)
- Red wine (in moderation)

Miscellaneous
- Gluten-free baking flour (almond flour, coconut flour)
- Gluten-free pasta (brown rice pasta, quinoa pasta)
- Organic bone broth
- Fresh herbs (cilantro, parsley, basil)

Baking Staples
Anti-Inflammatory, Low Sugar & Gluten-Free

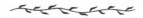

These staples will help you create a variety of delicious and healthy baked goods that align with an anti-inflammatory, low-sugar, and gluten-free meal plan.

Flours and Grains
- Almond flour
- Coconut flour
- Gluten-free oat flour
- Cassava flour
- Buckwheat flour
- Quinoa flour
- Lupin flour
- Arrowroot powder (for thickening and as a flour alternative)

Sweeteners
- Stevia (powder or liquid)
- Monk fruit sweetener
- Coconut sugar (in moderation, lower glycemic index)
- Pure maple syrup (in moderation)
- Raw honey (in moderation)

Leavening Agents
- Baking soda (aluminum-free)
- Baking powder (gluten-free, aluminum-free)
- Cream of tartar

Binders and Thickeners
- Flaxseed meal (for flax eggs, thickening)
- Chia seeds (for chia eggs, thickening)
- Psyllium husk powder (for adding structure and fiber)

- Xanthan gum (used sparingly for gluten-free baking)
- Agar-agar (a vegetarian gelatin alternative)

Healthy Fats and Oils
- Extra virgin olive oil (for savory baking)
- Coconut oil (solid or liquid)
- Avocado oil
- Ghee or clarified butter (for those who can tolerate dairy)
- Nut butters (almond butter, cashew butter)

Spices and Flavorings
- Cinnamon
- Nutmeg
- Ginger
- Turmeric
- Vanilla extract (pure, alcohol-free if possible)
- Almond extract

Dairy and Diary Alternatives
- Unsweetened almond milk
- Unsweetened coconut milk
- Full-fat Greek yogurt (for adding moisture and protein)
- Coconut cream (for rich, dairy-free alternatives)
- Dairy-free chocolate chips (dark chocolate, low in sugar)

Nuts, Seeds, and Add-ins
- Raw nuts: almonds, walnuts, pecans, hazelnuts
- Seeds: pumpkin seeds, sunflower seeds, sesame seeds
- Shredded unsweetened coconut
- Dried fruit (unsweetened, in moderation): dates, raisins, cranberries
- Dark chocolate: 70% cocoa or higher, chopped or as chips
- Collagen peptides (for protein and structure in baked goods)

Miscellaneous
- Gluten-free baking powder
- Gelatin (for binding in gluten-free recipes)
- Sea salt or Himalayan pink salt
- Apple cider vinegar (used in some recipes for leavening)

Breakfast Recipes

These breakfast meals are nutritious, flavorful, and aligned with the principles of the REBOOT, ensuring a healthy start to your day while keeping sugar and gluten at bay.

1. **Greek Yogurt Parfait**

   Ingredients:
   - 1 cup plain Greek yogurt
   - 1/2 cup mixed berries (blueberries, raspberries, strawberries)
   - 1 tablespoon chia seeds
   - 1 tablespoon chopped nuts (almonds or walnuts)
   - A drizzle of honey (optional, for extra sweetness)

   Instructions:
   - Layer the Greek yogurt in a bowl
   - Top with mixed berries, chia seeds, and chopped nuts
   - Drizzle with honey if desired

2. **Veggie Omelette**

   Ingredients:
   - 2-3 eggs, scrambled
   - 1/4 cup chopped spinach
   - 1/4 cup diced tomatoes
   - 1/4 cup diced bell peppers
   - 1/4 cup crumbled feta cheese
   - 1 tablespoon olive oil
   - Salt and pepper to taste

   Instructions:
   - Heat olive oil in a skillet over medium heat.

- Add the spinach, tomatoes, and bell peppers, and sauté until soft.
- Pour the beaten eggs over the vegetables and cook until the eggs are set.
- Sprinkle with feta cheese and fold the omelette.
- Season with salt and pepper to taste.

3. Avocado Toast on Sweet Potato Slices

Ingredients:
- 1 large sweet potato, sliced into 1/4-inch thick pieces
- 1 ripe avocado
- 1 tablespoon lemon juice
- Salt and pepper to taste
- Optional toppings: cherry tomatoes, radishes, micro-greens

Instructions:
- Toast the sweet potato slices in a toaster or bake in the oven at 400°F (200°C) for about 20 minutes, flipping halfway through.
- Mash the avocado in a bowl and mix with lemon juice, salt, and pepper.
- Spread the mashed avocado on the toasted sweet potato slices.
- Add optional toppings like cherry tomatoes, radishes, or micro-greens.

4. Anti-Inflammatory Quinoa Breakfast Bowl with Eggs

Ingredients:
- 1/2 cup cooked quinoa
- 1 large egg, poached or soft-boiled
- 1/2 avocado, sliced
- 1/4 cup steamed or sautéed spinach
- 1/4 cup roasted sweet potatoes, diced

- 1 tablespoon ground flaxseeds or chia seeds
- 1 tablespoon pumpkin seeds (pepitas)
- 1 teaspoon turmeric powder (for extra anti-inflammatory benefits)
- 1 tablespoon olive oil
- 1 tablespoon apple cider vinegar
- Salt and pepper to taste

Instructions:
- Prepare the Quinoa: Cook the quinoa according to package instructions. Let it cool slightly.
- Cook the Egg: Poach or soft-boil the egg.
- Assemble the Bowl: In a bowl, start with the cooked quinoa as your base. Arrange the sliced avocado, steamed spinach, and roasted sweet potatoes on top.
- Add Seeds and Spices: Sprinkle the ground flaxseeds, pumpkin seeds, and turmeric over the top.
- Dress the Bowl: Drizzle with olive oil and apple cider vinegar. Season with salt and pepper to taste.
- Top with Egg: Place the poached or soft-boiled egg on top.
- Serve: Enjoy this hearty, nutritious breakfast bowl that's packed with anti-inflammatory ingredients to start your day right!

5. *Mediterranean Smoothie*

Ingredients:
- 1 cup unsweetened almond milk
- 1/2 cup Greek yogurt
- 1 cup spinach
- 1/2 cup frozen berries (blueberries, raspberries, strawberries)
- 1 tablespoon chia seeds

- 1 tablespoon almond butter

Instructions:
- Combine all ingredients in a blender.
- Blend until smooth and creamy.
- Pour into a glass and enjoy.

6. *Cottage Cheese Protein Pancakes with Mixed Berries*

Ingredients:
- 1 cup almond flour
- 1/2 cup cottage cheese
- 2 large eggs
- 1/4 cup unsweetened almond milk (or any other dairy-free milk)
- 1 tablespoon coconut oil, melted
- 1 teaspoon vanilla extract
- 1/2 teaspoon baking powder
- A pinch of salt
- 1 scoop of vanilla protein powder (whey, plant-based, or collagen protein)
- 1 tablespoon ground flaxseeds (optional for extra fiber)
- 1/2 cup mixed berries (e.g., blueberries, raspberries, blackberries)
- Coconut oil or butter for cooking

Instructions:
- Mix the Batter: In a blender or mixing bowl, combine the almond flour, cottage cheese, eggs, almond milk, melted coconut oil, vanilla extract, protein powder, baking powder, ground flaxseeds, and salt. Blend or whisk until the batter is smooth and well combined. The batter should be thick but pourable.

- Cook the Pancakes: Heat a non-stick skillet over medium heat and lightly grease with coconut oil or butter. Pour about 1/4 cup of batter onto the skillet for each pancake. Cook until bubbles form on the surface and the edges start to look set, then flip and cook for another 1-2 minutes until golden brown.

- Add Berries: Once the pancakes are cooked, top them with your choice of mixed berries. Alternatively, you can fold the berries into the batter just before cooking.

- Serve: Serve the pancakes warm, with a dollop of Greek yogurt or a drizzle of pure maple syrup if desired, though keep in mind this will add some sugar.

Note: _If you're looking for even more protein, you can add an extra scoop of protein powder or serve with a side of scrambled eggs (or egg whites). Keep these pancakes low-sugar by sticking to the berries and avoiding additional sweetness._

7. *Mediterranean Turkey Bacon and Veggie Scramble*
    Ingredients:
    - 2 slices turkey bacon
    - 2 large eggs
    - 1/4 cup cherry tomatoes, halved
    - 1/4 cup chopped spinach
    - 1/4 bell pepper, diced
    - 1 tablespoon red onion, diced
    - 1 tablespoon crumbled feta cheese (optional)
    - 1 tablespoon extra virgin olive oil
    - Salt and pepper to taste
    - Fresh herbs like parsley or basil for garnish

Instructions:
- Cook the Turkey Bacon: Heat a non-stick skillet over medium heat and cook the turkey bacon until crispy. Remove from the pan and set aside.
- Prepare the Veggies: In the same skillet, add the olive oil and sauté the red onion and bell pepper for 2-3 minutes until softened.
- Add the cherry tomatoes and spinach, cooking until the spinach is wilted.
- Make the Scramble: In a small bowl, whisk the eggs with a pinch of salt and pepper. Pour the eggs into the skillet with the veggies, stirring gently to scramble them.
- Combine and Serve: Chop the cooked turkey bacon into bite-sized pieces and stir it into the egg scramble. Sprinkle with crumbled feta cheese, if using, and garnish with fresh herbs.
- Serve immediately with a side of fresh fruit or a small salad.

This turkey bacon and veggie scramble is a delicious and protein-packed breakfast that's low in sugar, gluten-free, and fits perfectly into an anti-inflammatory meal plan.

Lunch Recipes

These recipes are flavorful, nutritious, and align with the REBOOT principles, making them perfect for a healthy and satisfying lunch.

1. ***Quinoa and Chickpea Salad***
   Ingredients:
   - 1 cup quinoa, cooked and cooled
   - 1 can chickpeas, drained and rinsed
   - 1 cucumber, diced
   - 1 bell pepper, diced
   - 1/2 red onion, finely chopped
   - 1/4 cup chopped fresh parsley
   - 1/4 cup crumbled feta cheese
   - Juice of 1 lemon
   - 2 tablespoons extra virgin olive oil
   - Salt and pepper to taste

   Instructions:
   - In a large bowl, combine the quinoa, chickpeas, cucumber, bell pepper, red onion, parsley, and feta cheese.
   - In a small bowl, whisk together the lemon juice, olive oil, salt, and pepper.
   - Pour the dressing over the salad and toss to combine.
   - Serve chilled or at room temperature.

Note: You can add a protein of choice, such as grilled chicken, tofu, or salmon

2. *Grilled Chicken and Vegetable Skewers*
   Ingredients:
   - 2 boneless, skinless chicken breasts, cut into chunks
   - 1 zucchini, sliced
   - 1 yellow squash, sliced
   - 1 red bell pepper, cut into chunks
   - 1 red onion, cut into chunks
   - 2 tablespoons extra virgin olive oil
   - Juice of 1 lemon
   - 2 cloves garlic, minced
   - 1 teaspoon dried oregano
   - Salt and pepper to taste

   Instructions:
   - In a bowl, combine olive oil, lemon juice, garlic, oregano, salt, and pepper.
   - Add the chicken and vegetables to the bowl and toss to coat.
   - Thread the chicken and vegetables onto skewers.
   - Grill over medium-high heat for 10-12 minutes, turning occasionally, until the chicken is cooked through and the vegetables are tender.
   - Serve with a side of tzatziki sauce if desired.

3. *Mediterranean Stuffed Bell Peppers*
   Ingredients:
   - 4 bell peppers, tops cut off and seeds removed
   - 1 cup cooked quinoa
   - 1 can black beans, drained and rinsed
   - 1/2 cup diced tomatoes
   - 1/4 cup chopped Kalamata olives
   - 1/4 cup crumbled feta cheese
   - 2 tablespoons chopped fresh basil
   - 1 tablespoon extra virgin olive oil

- Salt and pepper to taste

Instructions:
- Preheat oven to 375°F (190°C).
- In a large bowl, combine the quinoa, black beans, tomatoes, olives, feta cheese, basil, olive oil, salt, and pepper.
- Stuff the bell peppers with the quinoa mixture.
- Place the stuffed peppers in a baking dish and cover with foil.
- Bake for 30 minutes, then remove the foil and bake for an additional 10-15 minutes, until the peppers are tender.
- Serve hot

4. Spinach and Feta Stuffed Portobello Mushrooms

Ingredients:
- 4 large Portobello mushrooms, stems removed
- 2 cups fresh spinach, chopped
- 1/2 cup crumbled feta cheese
- 1/4 cup chopped sun-dried tomatoes (not in oil)
- 2 cloves garlic, minced
- 2 tablespoons extra virgin olive oil
- Salt and pepper to taste

Instructions:
- Preheat oven to 400°F (200°C).
- In a skillet, heat 1 tablespoon of olive oil over medium heat. Add the garlic and spinach, and cook until the spinach is wilted.
- Remove from heat and stir in the feta cheese and sun-dried tomatoes.
- Brush the mushroom caps with the remaining olive oil and season with salt and pepper.
- Place the mushrooms on a baking sheet and fill each with the spinach mixture.

- Bake for 20-25 minutes, until the mushrooms are tender and the filling is heated through.
- Serve hot.

5. *Mediterraean Tuna Salad Lettuce Wraps*

Ingredients
- 1 can tuna in olive oil, drained
- 1/2 cup diced cucumber
- 1/2 cup diced tomatoes
- 1/4 cup diced red onion
- 1/4 cup chopped Kalamata olives
- 2 tablespoons chopped fresh parsley
- 2 tablespoons extra virgin olive oil
- Juice of 1 lemon
- Salt and pepper to taste
- Large lettuce leaves (such as Romaine or Bibb), for wrapping

Instructions:
- In a large bowl, combine the tuna, cucumber, tomatoes, red onion, olives, and parsley.
- In a small bowl, whisk together the olive oil, lemon juice, salt, and pepper.
- Pour the dressing over the tuna mixture and toss to combine.
- Spoon the tuna salad onto large lettuce leaves and wrap them up.
- Serve immediately.

6. *Mediterranean Chicken Salad with Spinach and Avocado*

Ingredients:
- 2 boneless, skinless chicken breasts
- 4 cups fresh baby spinach
- 1 avocado, sliced
- 1/2 cup cherry tomatoes, halved
- 1/4 cup red onion, thinly sliced

- 1/4 cup Kalamata olives, pitted and halved
- 1/4 cup crumbled feta cheese
- 2 tablespoons extra virgin olive oil
- Juice of 1 lemon
- 1 teaspoon dried oregano
- Salt and pepper to taste

Instructions:

- Cook the Chicken: Season the chicken breasts with salt, pepper, and dried oregano. Heat 1 tablespoon of olive oil in a skillet over medium-high heat. Cook the chicken for 6-7 minutes per side, or until cooked through. Remove from the skillet and let rest for a few minutes, then slice into strips.
- Prepare the Salad: In a large salad bowl, combine the baby spinach, sliced avocado, cherry tomatoes, red onion, olives, and crumbled feta cheese.
- Dress the Salad: In a small bowl, whisk together the remaining olive oil and lemon juice. Season with salt and pepper to taste.
- Assemble and Serve: Add the sliced chicken to the salad. Drizzle with the lemon-olive oil dressing and toss to combine. Serve immediately.

7. *Mediterranean Stuffed Avocados*

Ingredients:

- 2 large ripe avocados, halved and pitted
- 1 can (5 oz) tuna in olive oil, drained
- 1/4 cup cherry tomatoes, diced
- 1/4 cup cucumber, diced
- 2 tablespoons red onion, finely chopped
- 1/4 cup Kalamata olives, pitted and chopped
- 2 tablespoons fresh parsley, chopped
- 1 tablespoon extra virgin olive oil
- Juice of 1 lemon

- Salt and pepper to taste

Instructions:
- Prepare Tuna Mixture: In a medium bowl, combine the drained tuna, cherry tomatoes, cucumber, red onion, olives, and parsley.
- Dress the Mixture: Add the olive oil and lemon juice to the tuna mixture, and season with salt and pepper. Toss to combine.
- Stuff Avocados: Spoon the tuna mixture into the hollowed-out centers of the avocado halves.
- Serve: Serve immediately as a light and refreshing lunch.

Dinner Recipes

These recipes are flavorful, nutritious, and align with the REBOOT meal plan principles, making them perfect for a healthy, anti-inflammatory, and gluten-free dinner.

1. ***Lemon Herb Grilled Salmon with Quinoa and Asparagus***
   Ingredients:
   - 4 salmon fillets
   - 2 tablespoons extra virgin olive oil
   - Juice of 2 lemons
   - 2 cloves garlic, minced
   - 1 teaspoon dried oregano
   - Salt and pepper to taste
   - 1 cup quinoa, rinsed
   - 2 cups water or vegetable broth
   - 1 bunch asparagus, trimmed

   Instructions:
   - Marinate the Salmon: In a small bowl, whisk together olive oil, lemon juice, garlic, oregano, salt, and pepper. Pour over salmon fillets and let marinate for at least 30 minutes.
   - Cook Quinoa: In a medium saucepan, bring water or vegetable broth to a boil. Add quinoa, reduce heat, cover, and simmer for 15 minutes or until liquid is absorbed. Fluff with a fork.
   - Grill Asparagus: Toss asparagus with a little olive oil, salt, and pepper. Grill or roast at 400°F (200°C) for 10-15 minutes until tender.
   - Grill Salmon: Preheat grill to medium-high heat. Grill salmon for about 4-5 minutes per side, or until cooked through.
   - Serve: Plate the salmon with quinoa and asparagus on the side. Garnish with fresh lemon slices and herbs if desired.

2. *Mediterranean Chicken and Vegetable Bake*
   Ingredients:
   - 4 boneless, skinless chicken breasts
   - 1 zucchini, sliced
   - 1 yellow squash, sliced
   - 1 red bell pepper, sliced
   - 1 red onion, sliced
   - 1/4 cup Kalamata olives, pitted and halved
   - 2 tablespoons extra virgin olive oil
   - 2 cloves garlic, minced
   - 1 teaspoon dried basil
   - 1 teaspoon dried oregano
   - Salt and pepper to taste
   - 1/4 cup crumbled feta cheese

   Instructions:
   - Preheat Oven: Preheat oven to 400°F (200°C).
   - Prepare Vegetables: In a large baking dish, combine zucchini, squash, bell pepper, onion, and olives. Drizzle with olive oil and season with garlic, basil, oregano, salt, and pepper. Toss to coat.
   - Add Chicken: Nestle the chicken breasts into the vegetables.
   - Bake: Bake for 25-30 minutes, or until the chicken is cooked through and the vegetables are tender.
   - Serve: Sprinkle with feta cheese before serving.

3. *Shrimp and Avocado Salad*
   Ingredients:
   - 1 lb shrimp, peeled and deveined
     2 tablespoons extra virgin olive oil
   - Juice of 1 lime
   - 2 cloves garlic, minced
   - Salt and pepper to taste
   - 2 avocados, diced
   - 1 cucumber, diced
   - 1 cup cherry tomatoes, halved
   - 1/4 cup red onion, finely chopped

- 1/4 cup fresh cilantro, chopped

Instructions:
- Marinate Shrimp: In a bowl, combine olive oil, lime juice, garlic, salt, and pepper. Add shrimp and marinate for 15-20 minutes.
- Cook Shrimp: Heat a skillet over medium-high heat. Add shrimp and cook for 2-3 minutes per side, or until pink and opaque. Remove from heat.
- Assemble Salad: In a large bowl, combine avocado, cucumber, cherry tomatoes, red onion, and cilantro. Add cooked shrimp and toss gently.
- Serve: Serve immediately, optionally with additional lime wedges.

4. *Eggplant and Tomato Stew*

Ingredients:
- 1 large eggplant, diced
- 1 can diced tomatoes (14.5 oz)
- 1 onion, chopped
- 2 cloves garlic, minced
- 1 red bell pepper, diced
- 2 tablespoons extra virgin olive oil
- 1 teaspoon dried oregano
- 1 teaspoon dried basil
- Salt and pepper to taste
- Fresh basil for garnish

Instructions:
- Prepare Eggplant: Place diced eggplant in a colander and sprinkle with salt. Let sit for 30 minutes to remove excess moisture. Rinse and pat dry.
- Cook Vegetables: In a large pot, heat olive oil over medium heat. Add onion and garlic, and sauté until softened. Add bell pepper and cook for another 5 minutes.
- Add Eggplant and Tomatoes: Add eggplant and cook for another 5 minutes. Stir in diced tomatoes, oregano, basil, salt, and pepper. Bring to a boil,

then reduce heat and simmer for 20-25 minutes, until vegetables are tender.
- Serve: Garnish with fresh basil before serving.

5. *Zucchini Noodles with Pesto and Grilled Chicken*
   Ingredients For the Zucchini Noodles:
   - 2 medium zucchinis (spiraled into noodles)
   - 2 boneless, skinless organic chicken breasts
   - 1 tablespoon extra virgin olive oil (for grilling chicken)
   - Sea salt and freshly ground black pepper to taste

   Ingredients For the Anti-Inflammatory Pesto:
   - 1 cup fresh basil leaves
   - 1/4 cup walnuts (anti-inflammatory alternative to pine nuts)
   - 1/4 cup nutritional yeast (or omit for a simpler pesto)
   - 2 cloves garlic
   - 1/4 cup extra virgin olive oil
   - Juice of 1/2 lemon (optional, for added anti-inflammatory benefits)
   - Sea salt and freshly ground black pepper to taste

   Instructions:
   - Prepare the Chicken: Season the chicken breasts with olive oil, sea salt, and freshly ground black pepper. Preheat a grill or grill pan over medium heat. Grill the chicken for 5-7 minutes per side, or until fully cooked and juices run clear. Remove from the grill and let the chicken rest for a few minutes before slicing it into thin strips.

   - Make the Anti-Inflammatory Pesto: In a food processor, combine the fresh basil leaves, walnuts, garlic, and lemon juice. Pulse until the ingredients are finely chopped.With the food processor running, slowly drizzle in the olive oil until the pesto reaches a smooth consistency. Season with sea salt and freshly ground black pepper to taste.

- Prepare the Zucchini Noodles: If you prefer raw zucchini noodles, you can skip this step or lightly sauté them in a large pan over medium heat for 1-2 minutes to soften them slightly. Be careful not to overcook them, as they can become mushy. Alternatively, enjoy the zucchini noodles raw for a fresher texture.

- Assemble the Dish: In a large bowl, toss the zucchini noodles with the prepared pesto until well coated. Divide the pesto-coated zucchini noodles between plates and top with the grilled chicken strips. Garnish with additional fresh basil or a sprinkle of nutritional yeast, if desired.

- Serve and Enjoy: Serve immediately while the chicken is still warm. Enjoy a light, flavorful meal that is rich in anti-inflammatory ingredients, low in sugar, and gluten-free.

6. *Baked Cod with Olive and Tomato Tapenade*
   Ingredients:
   - 4 cod fillets
   - 1/4 cup Kalamata olives, pitted and chopped
   - 1 cup cherry tomatoes, halved
   - 2 cloves garlic, minced
   - 2 tablespoons capers, drained
   - 2 tablespoons extra virgin olive oil
   - 1 tablespoon fresh parsley, chopped
   - Juice of 1 lemon
   - Salt and pepper to taste
   Instructions:
   - Preheat Oven: Preheat oven to 375°F (190°C).
   - Prepare Tapenade:In a bowl, combine chopped olives, cherry tomatoes, garlic, capers, olive oil, parsley, lemon juice, salt, and pepper.

- Bake Cod: Place cod fillets in a baking dish and spoon the olive and tomato tapenade over the top. Bake for 15-20 minutes or until the fish is opaque and flakes easily with a fork.
- Serve: Serve immediately, garnished with additional parsley if desired.

7. *Greek-Style Stuffed Zucchini Boat*
   Ingredients:
   - 4 medium zucchinis
   - 1/2 pound ground turkey or beef
   - 1 small onion, finely chopped
   - 2 cloves garlic, minced
   - 1 cup diced tomatoes
   - 1/4 cup chopped Kalamata olives
   - 1/4 cup crumbled feta cheese
   - 2 tablespoons fresh parsley, chopped
   - 2 tablespoons extra virgin olive oil
   - Salt and pepper to taste

   Instructions:
   - Preheat Oven: Preheat oven to 375°F (190°C).
   - Prepare Zucchini: Slice zucchinis in half lengthwise and scoop out the seeds to create "boats."
   - Cook Filling: In a skillet, heat olive oil over medium heat. Add onion and garlic, and sauté until softened. Add ground turkey or beef and cook until browned. Stir in diced tomatoes, olives, salt, and pepper. Cook for another 5 minutes.
   - Stuff Zucchini: Place zucchini boats in a baking dish. Fill each boat with the meat mixture. Sprinkle with crumbled feta cheese.
   - Bake: Cover with foil and bake for 20 minutes. Remove the foil and bake for an additional 10 minutes or until the zucchini is tender.
   - Serve: Garnish with fresh parsley before serving.

Sweet Treats
Healthy, Protein-Rich, & Low Sugar

These recipes not only provide the delicious flavors and textures you enjoy but also give you an extra protein boost to support your dietary needs.

1. ### *Dark Chocolate Bark with Nuts & Seeds*
   <u>Ingredients:</u>
   - 1 cup dark chocolate (70% cocoa or higher), melted
   - 1-2 tablespoons low sugar protein powder (unflavored or chocolate-flavored)
   - 1/4 cup almonds, chopped
   - 1/4 cup walnuts, chopped
   - 1 tablespoon pumpkin seeds
   - 1 tablespoon sunflower seeds
   - A pinch of sea salt

   <u>Instructions:</u>
   - Line a baking sheet with parchment paper.
   - Mix the protein powder into the melted dark chocolate.
   - Pour the chocolate onto the parchment paper, spreading it evenly.
   - Sprinkle the chopped nuts and seeds over the chocolate.
   - Add a pinch of sea salt on top.
   - Refrigerate for about 30 minutes, or until the chocolate is firm.
   - Break into pieces and enjoy.

2. Chia Seed Pudding

Ingredients:
- 1/4 cup chia seeds
- 1 cup unsweetened almond milk (or coconut milk)
- 1 scoop low sugar protein powder (vanilla or unflavored)
- 1-2 teaspoons stevia or monk fruit sweetener (to taste)
- 1/2 teaspoon vanilla extract
- Fresh berries (optional topping)
- A handful of nuts or a dollop of Greek yogurt (optional for extra protein)

Instructions:
- In a bowl or jar, mix the almond milk, protein powder, chia seeds, sweetener, and vanilla extract.
- Stir well to ensure everything is evenly distributed.
- Cover and refrigerate for at least 4 hours or overnight.
- Top with fresh berries and additional nuts or Greek yogurt before serving.

3. Almond Flour Cookies

Ingredients:
- 2 cups almond flour
- 1/4 cup coconut oil, melted
- 1/4 cup monk fruit sweetener
- 1/4 cup low sugar protein powder (vanilla or unflavored)
- 1 teaspoon vanilla extract
- 1/2 teaspoon baking soda
- A pinch of salt
- Optional: 1/4 cup dark chocolate chips
- 1 extra egg white (optional for even more protein)

Instructions:
- Preheat your oven to 350°F (175°C) and line a baking sheet with parchment paper.
- In a bowl, mix the almond flour, protein powder, sweetener, baking soda, and salt.
- Add the melted coconut oil, vanilla extract, and egg white, stirring until a dough forms.
- If using, fold in the dark chocolate chips.
- Scoop the dough into small balls and place them on the baking sheet, flattening them slightly.
- Bake for 10-12 minutes, or until the edges are golden brown.
- Let cool before enjoying.

4. *Avocado Chocolate Mousse*

Ingredients:
- 2 ripe avocados, peeled and pitted
- 1/4 cup unsweetened cocoa powder
- 1/4 cup almond milk
- 1/4 cup Greek yogurt or 1 scoop low sugar protein powder (chocolate or unflavored)
- 2-3 tablespoons stevia or monk fruit sweetener (to taste)
- 1 teaspoon vanilla extract

Instructions:
- Place the avocados, cocoa powder, almond milk, Greek yogurt or protein powder, sweetener, and vanilla extract in a blender or food processor.
- Blend until smooth and creamy.
- Taste and adjust sweetness if needed.
- Chill in the refrigerator for at least 30 minutes before serving.

5. *Frozen Banana Bites*

Ingredients:

- 2 ripe bananas, sliced into rounds
- 1/2 cup dark chocolate (70% cocoa or higher), melted
- 1-2 tablespoons low sugar protein powder (vanilla or chocolate-flavored)
- 1 tablespoon chopped nuts (optional)
- 1 tablespoon shredded coconut (optional)

Instructions:

- Line a baking sheet with parchment paper.
- Mix the protein powder into the melted dark chocolate.
- Dip each banana slice into the chocolate, coating it evenly.
- Place the chocolate-covered banana slices on the baking sheet.
- Sprinkle with chopped nuts or shredded coconut if desired.
- Freeze for at least 1 hour before enjoying.

6. *Protein Balls*

Ingredients:

- 3/4 cup almond butter
- 1/4 cup coconut flour
- 2 tablespoons unsweetened shredded coconut
- 1 tablespoon chia seeds
- 1/4 cup low sugar protein powder (vanilla, chocolate, or unflavored)
- 2 tablespoons monk fruit sweetener (to taste)
- Optional: 1/4 cup dark chocolate chips
- 1/4 cup collagen peptides (optional for an extra protein boost)

<u>Instructions:</u>
- In a bowl, mix the almond butter, coconut flour, shredded coconut, chia seeds, protein powder, and sweetener until well combined.
- If using, fold in the dark chocolate chips and collagen peptides.
- Roll the mixture into small balls and place them on a plate or baking sheet.
- Refrigerate for at least 30 minutes before serving.

7. *Baked Apples*

<u>Ingredients:</u>
- 2 apples, cored
- 1/4 cup chopped nuts (e.g., walnuts, almonds)
- 2 tablespoons low sugar protein powder (vanilla or unflavored)
- 1 teaspoon cinnamon
- 1 tablespoon coconut oil
- Optional: 1 tablespoon raisins or unsweetened dried cranberries
- Greek yogurt or cottage cheese for serving (optional)

<u>Instructions:</u>
- Preheat your oven to 350°F (175°C).
- Place the cored apples in a baking dish.
- In a small bowl, mix the chopped nuts, low sugar protein powder, cinnamon, coconut oil, and optional dried fruit (no added sugar).
- Stuff the mixture into the center of each apple.
- Bake for 20-25 minutes, or until the apples are tender.
- Serve warm, optionally with a dollop of Greek yogurt or cottage cheese for added protein.

8. Lemon Coconut Energy Bites

Ingredients:
- 1 cup almond flour
- 1/2 cup unsweetened shredded coconut
- 2 tablespoons coconut oil, melted
- 1/4 cup protein powder (vanilla or unflavored)
- 1 tablespoon lemon zest
- 2-3 tablespoons lemon juice
- 2 tablespoons stevia or monk fruit sweetener (to taste)
- Optional: 1 tablespoon chia seeds or hemp seeds

Instructions:
- In a bowl, mix the almond flour, shredded coconut, low sugar protein powder, lemon zest, and sweetener.
- Add the melted coconut oil and lemon juice, stirring until the mixture comes together.
- If using, fold in the chia seeds or hemp seeds.
- Roll the mixture into small balls and place them on a plate or baking sheet.
- Refrigerate for at least 30 minutes before serving.

9. Ricotta Cheese with Cinnamon & Nuts

Ingredients:
- 1/2 cup ricotta cheese (full-fat, unsweetened)
- 1/4 cup Greek yogurt or cottage cheese
- 1/4 cup low sugar protein powder (vanilla or unflavored)
- 1/2 teaspoon cinnamon
- 1 tablespoon chopped nuts (e.g., almonds, walnuts)
- Optional: a few drops of vanilla extract or stevia for extra sweetness

Instructions:
- In a small bowl, mix the ricotta cheese, Greek yogurt or cottage cheese, protein powder, cinnamon, and vanilla extract or stevia if using.
- Top with chopped nuts.
- Serve immediately as a creamy and protein-rich snack.

High-Protein Snack Ideas
Low in Sugar & Gluten-free

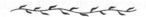

These snacks are quick to prepare and provide a satisfying, high-protein option that fits perfectly within an anti-inflammatory lifestyle. They are also low in sugar and gluten-free, making them ideal for a healthy, balanced lifestyle.

1. **Greek Yogurt with Nuts and Seeds**
   Ingredients:
   - 1 cup plain full-fat Greek yogurt
   - 1 tablespoon almonds or walnuts
   - 1 tablespoon chia seeds

2. **Hummus and Veggie Sticks**
   Ingredients:
   - 1/4 cup hummus
   - Carrot sticks, cucumber slices, and/or bell pepper slices

3. **Turkey Roll-Ups**
   Ingredients:
   - 3-4 slices of turkey breasts
   - 1/4 avocado
   - 1 tablespoon dijon mustard
   - A few spinach leaves

4. **Tuna Salad on Cucumber Slices**
   Ingredients:
   - 1 small can of tuna (packed in water)
   - 1 tablespoon olive oil
   - Lemon juice
   - Cucumber slices
   - Salt and pepper to taste

5. Boiled Eggs with Olive Tapenade
Ingredients:
- 2 boiled eggs
- 1 tablespoon olive tapenade

6. Cottage Cheese with Pine Nuts and Tomatoes
Ingredients:
- 1/2 cottage cheese
- 1 tablespoon pine nuts
- Cherry tomatoes
- Drizzle of olive oil

7. Smoked Salmon and Avocado Bites
Ingredients:
- 2 slices smoked salmon
- 1/2 avocado
- 1 teaspoon lemon juice
- A few dill springs

8. Almond Butter and Apple Slices
Ingredients:
- 1 splice, sliced
- 2 tablespoons almond butter

9. Edamame with Sea Salt
Ingredients:
- 1 cup shelled edamame (boiled or steamed)
- Pinch of sea salt

10. Chickpea Salad with Feta
Ingredients:
- 1/2 cup canned chickpeas (rinsed and drained)
- 1 tablespoon crumbled feta cheese
- 1 tablespoon olive oil
- A squeeze of lemon juice
- Salt and pepper to taste

Grab-and-Go Healthy Snacks
Low in Sugar & Anti-Inflammatory

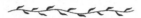

These snacks are easy to grab and take on the go, providing anti-inflammatory benefits while being low in sugar. They are also nutrient-dense, helping to keep you satisfied between meals.

1. *Raw Nuts and Seeds:* Almonds, walnuts, cashews, pistachios, pumpkin seeds, sunflower seeds

2. *Fresh Fruit:* Berries (blueberries, strawberries, raspberries), splice slices, pear slices, oranges or tangerines, grapes

3. *Veggie Sticks with Hummus:* Carrot sticks, celery sticks, cucumber slices, bell pepper slices

4. *Hard-Boiled Eggs:* Ready-to-eat, packed with protein and healthy fats

5. *Avocado Slices or Guacamole Cups:* Pair with veggie sticks or enjoy on its own

6. *Dark Chocolate (70% cocoa or higher):* A small piece of satisfies cravings and provides antioxidants

7. *Nut Butter Packets:* Almond butter or cashew butter (look for no added sugar), pair with an apple or celery sticks

8. *Olives:* Pre-packaged or from a jar, rich in healthy fats

9. *Chia Seed Pudding (pre-made or homemade):* Made with unsweetened almond milk and chia seeds, lightly sweetened with stevia or monk fruit

10. *Roasted chickpeas:* Crunchy, high-protein snack seasoned with anti-inflammatory spices like turmeric or paprika

11. *Cottage Cheese or Greek Yogurt (Full-fat, plain):* Add a handful of fresh berries or a sprinkle of nuts for extra flavor

12. *Seaweed Snacks:* Light, crunchy, and full of minerals

13. *Edamame:* Steamed and lightly salted, rich in protein and fiber

14. *Trail Mix (Homemade or Low-Sugar Store Bought):* Mix of raw nuts, seeds, and a few unsweetened dried fruits like cranberries or goji berries

15. *Protein Bars (Low-sugar, anti-inflammatory ingredients):* Look for bars made with whole foods, nuts, seeds, and minimal added sugars (no more than 5g added sugar)

Made in the USA
Monee, IL
12 November 2024

69957402R00095